D0823101

Will There Be Cows In Heaven?

Finding the "ancer" in cancer

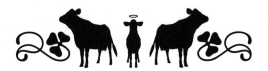

Will There Be Cows In Heaven?

Finding the "ancer" in cancer

Give GLORY to your story.

MARY E. MATTHIAS

FOREWORD BY H. MARSHALL MATTHEWS, MD

Mary Matthias

Two Harbors Press

Minneapolis

Copyright © 2009 by Mary E. Matthias. All rights reserved.

Two Harbors Press
212 3rd Avenue North, Suite 290
Minneapolis, MN 55401
612.455.2293
www.TwoHarborsPress.com

All rights reserved. No part of this publication may be reproduced, stored in a retrieval system, or transmitted, in any form or by any means, electronic, mechanical, photocopying, recording, or otherwise, without the written prior permission of the author.

ISBN - 978-1-935097-67-9
ISBN - 1-935097-67-9
LCCN - 2009941122

Cover Design and Typeset by Kristeen Wegner

Printed in the United States of America

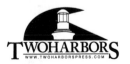

I Just Wanted to Be Sure of You

To Meg, my womb mate and my soul mate,
for all the times that you took my hand
and walked me through the storms.

Piglet sidled up to Pooh from behind,
"Pooh!" he whispered. "Yes, Piglet?"
"Nothing," said Piglet, taking Pooh's paw.
"I just wanted to be sure of you."
~~A.A. Milne

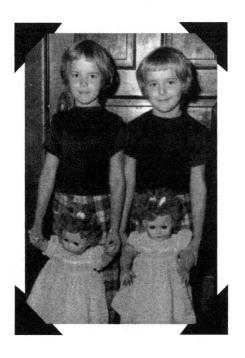

Contents

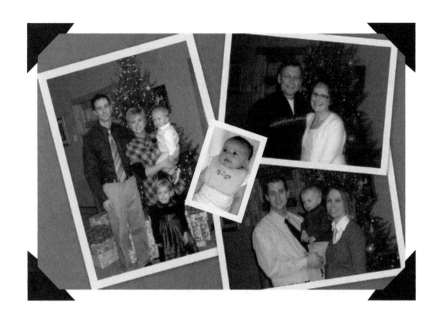

Thankfulness

"It sighs in satisfaction over a humble task done to God's glory and exhilarates over a creative task completed."
~~Emilie Barnes

"We always thank God for all of you, mentioning you in our prayers."
~~1 Thessalonians 1:2

To my team of healthcare advocates: Dr. Mary Govier, Dr. Rodney Halvorsen, Dr. Mansoor Shariff, Dr. H. Marshall Matthews, humble and heart-felt gratitude for your wisdom, intuitiveness, expertise, and genuine compassion. Thank you for embracing me and my family during some electrifying and defying times. Thank you for your God-directed guidance throughout my journey and for your ongoing love and support. Above all, thank you for your spirit of celebration in my grace-filled moments.

I am grateful to my friends and fellow Fork Ladies who have cried with me, carried me, and held me. Thank you for your many labors of love and for your healing words. To my many prayer warriors, those who donated ETO and other gifts, wore "Mary Ribbons," and made my Grand Canyon dream trip come true, I will never forget your gracious generosity! To all those who contributed in giving me an upstairs bathroom...you rock! To those of you who visited pity city with me but then showed me the way back to life's playground...gracias! To all of my caregivers, chauffeurs, cooks, cleaners, and chemo partners, you made such a difference in my life. Most of all, thank you for remaining at my side through times of adversity and for being there to celebrate my many milestones. You truly are earth angels.

To my Cancer Care Center Comrades, thank you for accompanying me on the roller coaster of life. It's been quite a ride. Your support, encouragement, humor, and hugs are so appreciated. It is truly a blessing to work with each and every one of you.

Pastor Headrick and my St. John's family in Christ, my family is grateful for your loving support and humbled by your prayers of intercession. To feel the power of prayer in one's life is simply indescribable. God has graced me with abundant blessings...you are amongst them.

To my Riesterer and Matthias family members, thank you for unconditionally sharing the gifts of time, talent, and treasures...you lightened our load. It comforts me to know that you continue to walk beside me on a journey that knows no end.

Mark, Ryan, Angie, Luke, Kristin, Leah, Sam, Ben, Emily, Shawn, Angela, and Addison, you encompass my life with goodness and "grand-ness." You are my passion, my purpose, and the fuel that energizes me. You bring me great joy! How do I find the words to express my gratitude for continually encouraging me, supporting me, and believing in me? Thank you for your ongoing love, humor, and hugs. You have rallied with me and for me in the best of times and in the worst of times. Through the bittersweet, we have grown in faith and grown as a family. Our God is an awesome God!

To my husband—thank you for bringing my stories to life by gracing my pages with your passion for photography. To Sandy Adelman—without your knowledge and expertise, my binder would still be sitting on a shelf. To Randi Hetland—how can I ever thank you enough for constantly bugging me to write a book. You believed in me before I believed in myself.

Lastly, but of utmost significance, it is with sincere gratitude that I thank those who contributed to this book by giving me a story or an inspiration. What a privilege it is to "give them away where they are needed."

Foreword

~~ by H. Marshall Matthews, MD

This is *not* just any book about cancer. There are books about the diagnosis, the symptoms, and the types of cancer. There are books about the treatment of cancer. These books all serve an important purpose: the most compelling need for most people at the time of their initial diagnosis is to begin to understand their disease and begin to know what to do about their disease.

Then...suddenly...there is a realization for the individual with this new diagnosis of cancer, and for many of their family and friends surrounding them, their lives become completely different.

I will suggest to you that the diagnosis of cancer will rock almost everyone's spiritual foundation. It will seem hollow and patronizing for me to suggest that in the midst of something so dramatic, so life-changing, and perhaps devastating, there can be something good or fortunate. Much too often, the most important gifts of our lives are those that surround us every day but we miss until we face crisis. The weight of this book is not measured in ounces but in wisdom. It is heavily laden with Mary's insights, her reflections, and her spirituality, which will highlight those very gifts that can come to you or someone else in the darkest hours.

I have sat in the presence of many wonderful people whose lives have abruptly changed with the diagnosis of cancer. The depth and weight and uncertainty of the moment are sobering. It is easy for me as an oncologist to answer questions about the cancer itself or the treatment; but when all of these explanations are complete, it is obvious that most of us are left with even bigger questions and life quandaries. Why me? How can I go on like this? How can I bear this burden? How can I continue to find meaning in my life? Is this all that is left?

These are the most profound questions of all. The answers seem hidden and distant. Occasionally, there is an "angel in our midst" who helps light our path. Let Mary introduce you to your angel. The many overwhelming feelings that accompany the diagnosis of cancer include fear, hopelessness, and grief causing many to also feel helpless, desperate, and angry. There is a disabling sense of the complete loss of control. Many well-meaning people offer advice as to what direction to turn. The most helpful voices usually arise from those who have taken the same journey. Mary has been on this journey.

Mary has a profound spirituality and faith. In her book she shares the observations of her own life experiences. In reflection, those observations offered her the very lessons she needed to survive the fear, the loss of control, and those subsequent feelings of hopelessness, anger, and grief. It is within this life review that the revelations occur that have allowed her to heal and move forward.

By paying attention to the gifts of each moment and the gifts of her most cherished memories, Mary is able to understand and immerse herself in the spirituality of her own life. Ironically, it is her darkest moment that has opened the door to allow her to see and feel and find those very things that she most needs to make sense of her life after her diagnosis of cancer. This, I believe, is what she needed most and what I suspect others need as well to support, heal, and nurture themselves in such a difficult experience. Mary's cancer experience reopened the door for her to pay attention. She has been able to weave together a series of beautiful observations that expose the universal tools for healing.

I cannot speak as a cancer survivor to the experiences that

Mary shares from her perspective of someone who "has been there." I try to astutely observe the experiences of those who are so kind as to allow me moments to share in some of the most personal aspects of their life. I can assure you that even in the midst of some of these most frightening and darkest moments I see unbelievable transformations of spirit, and these almost always occur along the lines of the messages that Mary brings to you.

~~ *H. Marshall Matthews, M.D.*

I Have a Story to Tell

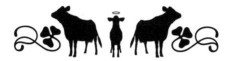

*"If stories come to you, care for them. And learn to give them away
where they are needed. Sometimes a person needs a story
more than food to stay alive. That is why we put these stories in
each other's memory. This is how people care for themselves.
One day you will be good story-tellers. Never forget these obligations."*
~~Barry Lopez
(as Badger, in Crow and Weasel)

In the children's book entitled *Crow and Weasel,* crow and weasel are
two fictional characters who venture out on a journey where they risk
death, gain wisdom, and eventually return home to share their stories.
Much like *Crow and Weasel,* I have been on a strikingly similar journey
yet vastly dissimilar. The difference being, I did not risk death but instead *death risked me.* If I am a wiser person because of it, it is merely
a consequence of my encounters along the way. By no means do I
claim to be a gifted story-teller; instead, I prefer to think of myself as
a story-gatherer. I believe that every one of us has a story worth telling
and worth receiving for all of life is full of moments worth gathering.
I have tenderly cared for these stories for the past 13 years; but before

I can give them away, there is something I must do. I need to return to where my journey began. An old proverb reads, "To know the road ahead, ask those coming back."

On May 29 1996, I began an arduous journey into a foreign land. Many times I did not know which path to take. I was lost, tired, and confused. I had no sense of direction, until I came to the intersection of HOPE. The curve in the road was called CANCER. At the age of 42, I went from being a caretaker to being taken care of. I was diagnosed with stage IIIa endometrial ovarian cancer. I will never forget the pain of coming home and telling my husband Mark and my two sons, Ryan age 17 and Luke age 14. I was quite adamant when I told them, "I am not planning on dying so don't you even begin to think that way." I had extensive surgery followed by six months of chemotherapy requiring three-four days of hospitalization at the time. Mission accomplished...end of journey...time to return home.

It was just two years later that I picked up the phone one evening and heard Dr. Matthew's voice. These were his words, "Mary, your tumor marker is up; and in my heart, I have been planning all day what we should do." Time to pack my HOPE bag and get on that road again! I was once again scheduled for a lengthy surgery which turned into a half hour open and closed procedure. The cancer was on my liver, on my diaphragm, and scattered all over my abdomen like confetti sprinkles. The physician came out of the operating room, took his mask off, and threw his arms up in the air. He told my husband, my sons, and my twin sister Meg, "The cancer has come back with vengeance. I am sorry there is nothing more that we can do for her." I was sent home to die or get my life in order, as he suggested. I went to Fleet Farm and bought big Rubbermaid totes and started to gather all that I ever wanted to share with my sons. I gathered pieces of their childhood, books, pictures, and stories. I wrote them love letters. I planned my funeral. I chose a new spouse for my husband to remarry. I prepared a living legacy. And I wept!

After about a month, Meg called me up and suggested, "Mary, you have done everything imaginable to prepare to die; and you will probably outlive us all, so why don't you come back to the living?" I proceeded to receive many more months of chemotherapy, and it is purely by the grace of God that I have been in remission for the past 11 years. I will always revere the Christmas that I sat with my sons and went through those totes together. The wisdom that I pass along in sharing this story is never let any earthly being stamp an expiration date on the bottom of your foot. Never let anyone destroy your hope. In Proverbs 24:14 we read, "Know also that wisdom is sweet to your soul; if you find it, there is future hope for you, and your hope will not be cut off."

When I was first diagnosed with cancer, I told Dr. Matthews that it was my hope to be a grandma one day; when, in reality, I was hoping to see my sons graduate from high school. Well my hope was certainly not cut off as I witnessed high school and college graduations. Dare I hope for more? It was with extreme elation that I witnessed my sons marry their beautiful life partners, Angie and Kristin. And the most "grand" gift of all...I am an Oma (Grandmother). God has filled our lives with the blessings of four grandchildren, Leah Rose, Samuel Jay, Benjamin Mark, and Emily June. Being an Oma simply humbles me to tears as it is a gift that has gone beyond my wildest expectations. I never asked God for it...it was simply given to me! I am in daily awe of His endless love.

Throughout my cancer treatment I had a personal mantra that became my daily chant, "Use me and help me to make a difference." I remember feeling very frustrated, as though I was a disappointment to God. I felt that if I didn't do great things with the time he graced me with that I would somehow be summoned home sooner. I found myself living life with such a sense of urgency. One day I shared these feelings with my pastor; and in his wisdom, he responded, "Mary, you don't have to get up on some band wagon or behind a podium. God gives us little opportunities each and every day. Use this time to do his greatest work...pray for others." And so I began a prayer journal and would pull it out while waiting in doctors' offices, while getting chemotherapy, or during those days when I had little energy to do anything more.

During my illness, I struggled professionally as a nurse. How could I nurture others when I was in desperate need of nurturing? I found myself physically and emotionally depleted with nothing left to give. I had lost all sense of compassion. I didn't even like who I was. Then one day someone cared so much about me that he stared into my lifeless and sunken eyes and said, "I am putting you on a one month leave of absence from your job, and you will not be going back. You need to figure it out." He knew what I needed at a time when I was so lost and confused (thank you Dr. Shariff). During my sabbatical from life, I counseled, I read, I took walks, I prayed, and I journaled.

May 19, 2002

"Almost six years since I was first diagnosed with cancer. Cancer has once again threatened to destroy my body, mind, and spirit. I am weary, broken, and trying to regain peace and harmony in my life. I hate cancer, but it does have its privileges. Cancer has allowed me to take a sabbatical from life. As I listen to my friends and family, I feel everyone could use at least a week away from the pace of the race. I am blessed that I have been given the wisdom, the resources, the tools, and the people to help me with this task. I needed to love myself again, for only then can you feel the love of others. I needed to feel the pain in order to feel the joy. I am starting to feel healthier, more energetic, more lighthearted, creative, and alive. I look at myself in the mirror, and I see peace returning and even a hint of sparkle in my eyes. What happened over these past few months? Why have I lost touch with my head, heart, and soul? How do I get it back? I'd like to blame it all on cancer; but in all actuality, I think I should be thanking cancer. I have been consumed by many earthly things. The uncertainty of my health is an ongoing balancing act. My life has been out of control; my head has been spinning. I have been fearful, sad, unable to concentrate, and physically ill. This week through "borrowed faith," prayer, and gentleness I have come to a renewed sense of peace. I have been so selfishly good to myself...a task that does not come easy, but I am learning to do it without guilt. Thank you God for allowing me to feel your arms wrapped so securely around me today." I wrote, *"I now know what I need to do."*

No, I was not given that epiphany moment in which I knew I must write a book—instead I was given a humbling opportunity to receive stories of joy and sadness, pain and passion, triumph and defeat from the inspiring people I was about to meet at Holy Family Memorial Cancer Care Center in Manitowoc, Wisconsin. Dr. Matthews expressed great concern about my own vulnerability and the emotional challenges of accepting this position. He did not want me to become "cancer consumed." I listened, I prayed on it, and then I remembered my mantra. I had to give it a try. I do find that my work requires an emotional balancing act especially during my own testing time. I also have to confess that it is never easy walking people to death's door, especially those who succumb to ovarian cancer! At times I suffer from an occasional bout of survivor's guilt which my comrades have helped me to work through. They repeatedly tell me that my work is not done and that God has plans for me. So instead of questioning why I am still alive, I simply embrace the mystery. It is humbling, and it is a privilege to share my story of hope to all of those who are beginning their own journey.

Since my cancer diagnosis, I have had the privilege of writing short stories for the Matthews Oncology Associates' supportive newsletter, TLC (Together we Live with Cancer) in which I have my own editorial called "Hope Happenings." The following stories are cumulative of those writings and are a sharing of my own personal journey with cancer as well as those that I have been gifted to receive. In the beginning, you may depict a sense of "rawness" in my early writings or perhaps better put, a sense of "aweness." In my 13 year journey with cancer, I have asked many questions: why me...what am I supposed to do with this...why not me? I just recently had a complete work-up and went to see Dr. Matthews with the grandiose illusion that perhaps after 13 years we could close the cancer book. I was told that I am in "uncharted territory."

What does that mean?

It means that I have time to explore.

I have found the "ancer" in cancer.

Stories have come to me,

I have cared for them,

And now I finally give them away...

For I have learned where they are needed!

M^cE M

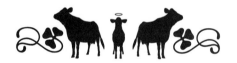

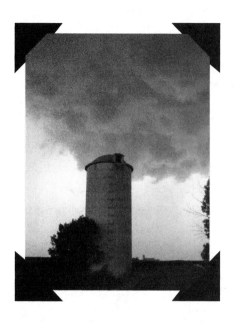

You Will Discover That You Have Two Hands

*I*n my work as a nurse, I am honored daily to meet some very extraordinary people. I took a liking to Charlie from the minute we first met. It was one of those rare encounters where our conversation flowed to a much deeper level all in a matter of 15 minutes. I have experienced relationships where I have *never* gotten to the level Charlie and I went to that day. It was like stopping at the home of a total stranger and being given a tour of the entire house from the basement all the way up to the attic. Charlie and I talked briefly about cancer, sharing our individual journeys with one another. We talked about prayer and the healing effect it had on both of our lives. We talked about having faith and trust in our physicians and in God. We talked about cancer being a life-altering experience. We shared with one another the ways in which it changed us personally. And then Charlie shared his soul.

He proceeded to tell me that he used to be a farmer; and whenever he was about to climb up his big old silo with those metal rungs that are spaced so far apart, he would pause and fold his hands together. He said that his farmer friends used to do the same thing, but there was one thing that he did differently. When his two feet were safely planted back on the soil, he would once again pause and fold his hands together. He told me that when he drives down Union Road and sees the baby eagles flapping their wings as they prepare to leave the nest, he pauses and says, "Thank you for giving me eyes to see." He went on to say that when he drives down Memorial Drive and hears the roaring white caps, he pauses and says, "Thank you for giving me ears to hear." And since cancer, every morning when he plants his feet on the ground, he pauses and says, "Thank you for giving me another day."

Charlie is a great storyteller and is very passionate about many things, including his love of cows. As I was leaving the exam room that day, Charlie looked at me ever so seriously. He said that he had a very important question to ask me…it has bothered him for some time; and if I did not have the answer, he hoped I could find out. Charlie quizzically pondered, "Do you think there will be cows in heaven?" I told Charlie that I thought there would not only be cows but eagles and roaring white caps too!

Thank-you Charlie for reminding me to always put my two hands together before I make that scary climb *and* when my feet are back on solid ground. Audrey Hepburn once said, "You will discover that you have two hands. One is for helping yourself and the other is for helping others." I think Charlie could quote it better, "You will discover that you have two hands when you learn how to bring them together."

Charlie is a wise and wonderful man. When I left the exam

room that day, I paused, put my hands together and said, "Thank-you for giving me a heart to receive...and please let there be cows in heaven."

We have one of those big old concrete silos with the metal runs right in our backyard. Before I sat down to write this story, I took a walk out there, paused, and folded my hands together. And thanks to Charlie's lesson, upon completion of writing, I repeated this ritual.

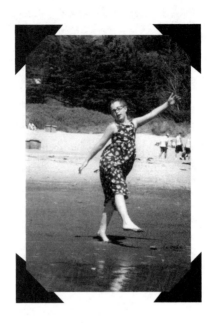

Free to Frolic

Do you find that certain words conjure up feelings that just make you smile? Recently my husband was trying to capture a picture of my friend and I amidst the butterflies in my flamboyant zinnia patch. Bette lightheartedly chimed, "Let's frolic!" The concept of frolicking brought a smile to my face; but admittedly, I had to stop and think. I needed to envision in my mind how a middle-aged woman should frolic. It felt awkward. Within the inhibitions of my adult mind, I felt certain that there was a rule prohibiting this. A warning sign went up in my head, "No one over the age of 50 should be allowed to frolic in the zinnia patch." Only children frolic through the leaves and the snow. Only a litter of puppies playfully frolic.

My godchild was visiting this summer, and she gave me a sequence of pictures of her dancing on the beach. She was unaware that her parents had captured her free spirit frolicking. I looked at that picture and longed to be a child again. I longed for the freedom to frolic on the beach. In the privacy of my home at that moment, I spread my arms and danced in my office. I felt clumsy and embarrassed. What if someone were to come walking in and find me frolicking in the middle of the afternoon? But I was now curious...why did it feel so good to frolic? How could I incorporate this foreign foolery back into my adult life? I have pondered this question for many weeks now making mental reminders to myself that I must remember to frolic. How can I possibly write about such experiences if I am not actively frolicking?

Last week I underwent some routine tests that raised some concerns about my cancer. I received a phone call at home from Dr. Matthews that my tumor markers were on the incline and that we needed to await CT results before deciding how to proceed. I was about to abort the idea of ever frolicking again until I received a phone call at work the next day saying that my CT scans were stable. Amidst tears, group hugs, and jumping up and down, I spread my arms and danced down the hall. I frolicked.

I have finally come to the realization that I have been frolicking all of my adult life. I have danced, laughed, played, joked, and celebrated. This summer I frolicked for 260 miles on the back of a Harley. What I have learned is that frolicking is not an activity but rather a state of mind. It is what enables us to celebrate life despite our limitations and adversities. It is what allows my soul the freedom to dance on the beach.

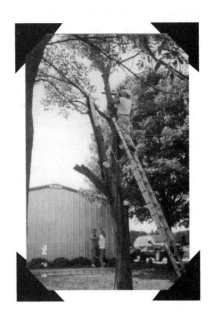

Remain Rooted

*I*n three short months, our 23 year old son Ryan will be married. Recently we invited him home for one last night as our son before he becomes Angie's husband. With great anticipation, we planned the evening in detail as we would for any special guest in our home. A big beautiful bouquet of flowers was picked from our yard. We prepared all of Ryan's favorite foods, dined by candlelight, and drank wine on our sun porch. Later that evening, Luke joined us around the bonfire for some reminiscing about our favorite family memories. That night as I turned down their beds, I savored the fact that this would probably be the last time my two sons would be present in that capacity.

The following morning began the big project of taking down

a grand old tree in our back yard–a storm had damaged it and it split down to the base. I watched as my husband and two sons stood back and planned their demolition strategy. As my three handsome lumberjacks stood there amidst the branches with chainsaws in hand, I ran for my camera. Finally the guys were getting a little irritated with me as I pleaded for them to stand still for "just one more picture." The work was rather precarious and required their concentration, so I decided to move indoors. I stood at my kitchen window and reflected on my vivid recall of two little boys climbing that grand old tree. As I took pictures with my pining heart, tears streamed down my cheeks. When did my little boys become young men? Later on that afternoon, feeling exhausted yet accomplished, my sons walked out the door with suitcases in hand. It has been a ponderous and emotional time for me since the events of that weekend. It was time to close another chapter in my life and search for the contents of a new beginning...or so I thought.

Over the next several weeks as I mourned my empty nest, I also mourned the loss of my grand old tree. I no longer had a place right by my kitchen window to hang my wind chimes and feed my beloved birds. I had to move my bench to a new shaded spot. But from there, I could no longer see the sunsets as I had in the past. Everything felt different; I longed for the familiarity of the past. One day as I sat on my newly repositioned bench, I gazed over at the remaining tree stump and considered this striking analogue. The sorrow that has been so deep rooted in my heart has not been for my sons...they are still very much a part of my life. It is not for my tree...we have many other grand old trees in our yard. The sorrow that I have felt comes from being storm damaged by cancer. I have been cracked, broken, weakened, and stripped of my leaves. Nothing in my life will ever be the same again. I long for the familiarity of my old life. I had been silently mourning my past.

What tragedy, disease, or loss causes your pining heart to

mourn? Remember there is one thing that no one can ever take away from you even when you are feeling as though you are cut down to nothing. Everything that you are stems from your roots. It is this system of values and beliefs that hopefully will keep my sons rooted in their past and future. There is no storm big enough that can ever destroy what lies buried within your heart and soul.

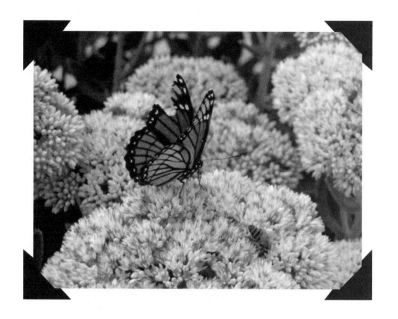

Flight to Freedom

*T*he butterfly started out to be a very important after death symbol for me but has now become a symbol of hope and personal growth. In a book entitled *Hello from Heaven,* authors Bill and Judy Guggenheim detail the phenomenon of After-Death Communication (ADC). "Some people are sent a sign spontaneously as a gift while others ask or pray to receive one. The receiver must interpret his or her own experience and assign personal meaning to it. The butterfly is a spiritual symbol of life after death because of its transformation from the caterpillar that crawls on the ground to the beautiful ethereal creature that flies through the air." Come fly with me as I share with you my butterfly blessings.

My mom was 64 years young when she succumbed to colon

cancer. As she lay in the hospital for three months physically deteriorating, I comforted my four year old and seven year old sons with a simple narrative. I explained to them that Grandma was like a cocoon, and one day soon out of that cocoon would come a beautiful butterfly...that would be Grandma's soul going to heaven. The day she died I came home, walked in the door, and said, "Guess what, Luke? Grandma is finally a butterfly!" He ran to his dad rejoicing, "Daddy, Daddy, it's the bestest day...Grandma is finally a butterfly." The next day I took my sons on a picnic lunch to a park. Imagine the awe when a butterfly landed on my knee. My mom became a butterfly epitaph.

At the age of 42 I was forced to face my own cancer diagnosis with a recurrence two years later. Following a tumor de-bulking surgery, I developed an illeus which, in layman's language, means that my bowel went to sleep. I was re-hospitalized with severe nausea, vomiting, and abdominal pain. I remember that night being the epitome of emotional and physical despair. An unsuccessful attempt was made to insert a tube into my stomach. At that point, my twin sister crawled into bed with me, held me in her arms, and prayed for a sign that everything would be okay. Imagine the awe once again when the entire TV screen was filled with a fluttering array of butterflies. To some it would have just been a Chevy commercial; but at that moment in time, the butterfly became my sign of hope and peace. God heard and answered our prayers on that dreadful night. At that point my vomiting ceased.

Just this past March, my 85 year old Dad was in critical care and had undergone surgery for a blocked carotid artery. As we were awaiting news from the surgeon, we decided to go to the cafeteria to pass some time. As we approached the elevator, there right in front of us was a beautiful picture of a butterfly with a poem of inspiration. Once again, such a sense of comfort and peace came over us with the appearance of this symbolic creature.

This past weekend we were invited to attend a wedding with a butterfly theme. I listened intently as I heard of the nurturing process that lead up to the gala butterfly release. Each guest was given a little white box, a message was read, and then everyone opened up their individual boxes as 200 butterflies fluttered to freedom...all but two that is. As two of these delicate creatures landed on the pavement, a gentle spirit came to their rescue. As he picked the butterflies up in his hand, he gave them each a little nudge sending them on their flight to freedom.

As I ponder this new butterfly phenomenon, I have assigned this beautiful ethereal creature final meaning. Have you ever felt like you were locked up in a cocoon? Is your spirit broken and your soul longing for transformation? What inhibits you from taking flight? I have learned many invaluable cancer lessons in the past six years. One of the most difficult is the art of surrendering. There have been many points in my life when I have fallen to the ground crying out in despair. Many times cancer has spun a cocoon around my life. I have felt like I could not escape. And then, a gentle spirit appears to pick me up, cradle me in his hands, and give me that little nudge to take flight. I am free at last. I am free to surrender, because I know that someone will always be there to pick me up. I am free to fly.

A Big Little Moment

Several weeks ago I became quite ill with a viral infection and possible bowel obstruction necessitating a visit to my friendly physician. Much to my chagrin, he proposed a hospital admission for dehydration. I drove myself back home, gathered some books and pajamas, and instructed my son what to prepare for dinner. I told him to tell his dad that I would be hanging out at the hospital for a few days in case he missed me. After two days, I was discharged home. On that day, they sent up a volunteer to escort me out the doors. He insisted that I go in a wheelchair and proceeded to ask me if someone was bringing the car around? I retorted, "That would be me." Somewhat puzzled and wanting to fulfill his duties as an escort, he insisted on wheeling me through the parking lot to my car. I really did not think it was a big deal...in fact, I thought it was quite comical. On my drive home that day, I got to thinking about this little event that had just transpired. What had emanated was a big, little moment in my life. It was my personal independence day.

On that special day I realized that my life was no longer a dictatorship ruled by cancer. I was reminiscent of the process. In *The Cancer Conqueror* by Greg Anderson, he says, "The medical community uses cancer as a noun. I encourage you to make cancer into a verb, an action verb. I challenge you to start to think, see, and feel yourself as *cancering.*" He further explains that "The verb *cancering* shifts our focus away from a disease we have and into the context of a process we are going through."

I have been *cancering* for six years now, and it certainly has been quite a process! In the beginning there was cancer, then there was cancer, and then there was even more cancer. That's all there was. I went into a survival mode, doing what I needed to do, and silently mourned the loss of my old, not so bad "normal" life. Remember, there are no laws or rules to govern how any of us should or should not respond in a life-altering experience. We must learn to respect where everyone is at in their life process. What I soon realized is that all of life is a continuous process of living and learning, longing and losing, with loving and laughing filling the spaces in between. In my process of *cancering* I have learned that it's the little moments filling the spaces in between that are bigger than life. I have learned that I can "live" with cancer.

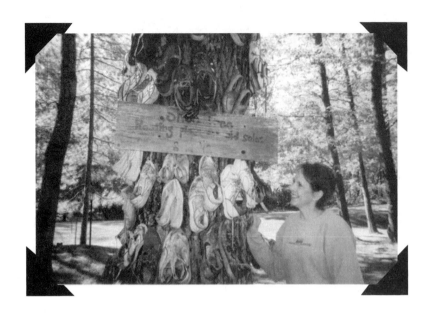

Hope Is...The Shoe Tree

*M*any treasured years ago my family and I vacationed at a cabin where we played together for a week. I will always remember our river rafting excursion as a day of mixed emotions. We started out our journey confident and full of energy. The river was unusually low that day. We got hung up on many rocks, lost an oar, and the falls were quite scary to unseasoned rafters. By mid-afternoon we were all weary, and I was near tears. Unfortunately, there's no turning back on a river. After many hours of struggling, we arrived safely at our destination. We felt such a feeling of accomplishment that night, so we celebrated by taking our shoes off and nailing them to a big old tree. We made a sign that read, "Shoe Tree...Resting Place for Old Soles." Our old shoe tree still stands strong to this day. It is adorned with a colorful variety of old shoes from other weary travelers who needed a place to rest their worn out soles.

My cancer journey has been much like my river journey. Many times I find myself getting hung up on rocks, going over frightening falls, and paddling upstream. Cancer has left me feeling weary, scared– like I'm about to drown. What do you do to repair your soul when it is all worn out? Take a "soul sabbatical." Learn to recognize when fear, worry, and stress is destroying your hope. Gather back that which saves you, re-define your hope, and find yourself a "shoe tree" to rest your weary soul upon. Flow with the river.

"Come to me, all who are weary and burdened,
And I will give you rest."
~~Matthew 11:28

Bless that Test

*N*ausea, insomnia, irritability, chest heaviness, loss of appetite, fatigue, inability to concentrate...with symptoms like these, one would think I should be seeking professional help. Actually these symptoms are quite normal, and I can predict when they are going to occur. I have diagnosed myself with pre-testing syndrome. It is a disease common to those who have been given a cancer diagnosis.

Five years ago, at the age of 42, I was diagnosed with ovarian cancer. My disease requires vigilant monitoring and frequent testing. Several weeks ago I experienced my first P.E.T. (Positron Emission Topography) scan at St. Vincent's in Green Bay. The good news about this high-tech procedure was that I didn't have to consume any unpalatable, thick milkshakes, and I got to keep my own clothes on. The bad news was I had to lie perfectly still for one hour after an injection was given. I was told not even to scratch myself or use my vocal chords. So they removed my husband and placed me on a slightly padded table behind a curtain to stare at the ceiling.

During that hour I tried desperately to not think about the itch I had on my leg or how badly I wanted to reposition myself. At one point a friend came in and started chitchatting and asking me questions. She was unaware that I was temporarily trapped inside my body. The only way I could communicate with her was to bat my eyes. It was during that hour that God gently reminded me of the abundant gifts of mind, body, and spirit that He daily endows my life with. He revealed to me the blessings amidst the adversity which I choose to call "hidden halos." That day I jumped off the exam table, verbalized my gratitude to Matt (the x-ray technician), and greeted my husband with a hug.

Relentless joy and gratitude, excessive energy, light-heartedness, insatiable appetite for life...I have just diagnosed myself with post-testing syndrome. Yes, I am still afraid; and I predict that in two months my symptoms will recur. But my hope has once again been fluffed up. *The Alpha Book on Cancer and Living* states, "Hope does not necessarily mean overcoming fear. It means feeling the presence of life even while you are afraid." Today, I lift my voice in praise of the good news I have been given. BLESS THAT TEST!

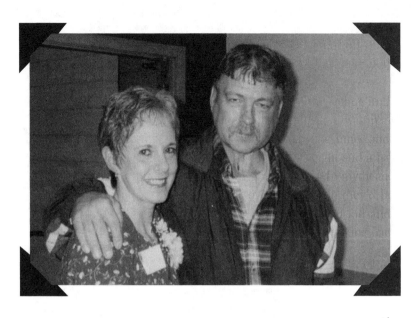

NCSD 2001 ♥ "Reflections"

Over the past few weeks I had the distinct delight of attending two NCSD (National Cancer Survivors Day) celebrations. This nation-wide event involves hundreds of communities and thousands of people across North America. For one day the world focuses on sur-vivorship issues. It is a day filled with tears, laughter, and lots of hugs. It is a time for survivors to come together to share stories of pain, courage, and hope.

The first event was the Matthew's Oncology "Hobby & Craft Showcase" held at the Knights of Columbus Hall in Sheboygan. As I stood behind my "Halo of Hope" card display in surveillance, I was overwhelmed with how alive the room felt and of the strong sense of camaraderie. I couldn't help but wonder if the secret to longevity is people who turn pain into passion. I was filled with *hopetimism* as people proudly displayed their years of survivorship on the name tags across their hearts. I also had the joy of meeting Matt, a very heroic 16 year old young man who has survived a brain tumor. I listened in awe and watched his face passionately glow as he spoke of his canoe trip to Canada right after chemo. I listened with deep admiration to his mother share her fears and concerns of this adventure at a time when Matt's white counts were very low. Thank you, Matt, for living out your dreams and for showing us that cancer cannot destroy our human spirits.

The second NCSD celebration I attended was a potluck lunch sponsored by the Holy Family Memorial Cancer Care Center in Manitowoc. This was truly a humbling and emotional experience for me as I was asked to share my own story of survivorship with my community. As we were being entertained by the Lincoln High School choral singers, I happened to notice a familiar face from my past walk through the doors. Six years ago I was a nurse for an ENT physician, and it was there that I first met Paul and his wife Sue. Paul was diagnosed in his thirties with cancer of the larynx and had to have his voice box removed. Paul faced many medical challenges after surgery, and he soon touched all of our hearts deeply with his warm smile and his gentle spirit. When I faced my second battle with ovarian cancer, Paul called me up and whispered into the phone, "You are going to beat this." That day as I stepped away from the podium, he met me with a warm hug and tears streaking down his cheeks. He once again whispered in my ear. "You know why I am here today? I am here for you because you were always there for me." I started to sob as I realized that he wasn't there because he is a survivor, but he was there to support me. We continued to hug and cry as his wife snapped pictures of the two of us. Thank you, Paul, for living and loving so unselfishly. Thank you for reminding us to listen to life's gentle whisperings.

What is a survivor? From the day you are diagnosed with cancer, you are a survivor. Being a survivor means *"being"* alive, not *"staying"* alive. How does one *"be"* alive while living with a life-threatening disease? You keep dreaming, live passionately, and love selflessly. Thanks for the bittersweet memories of NCSD 2001!

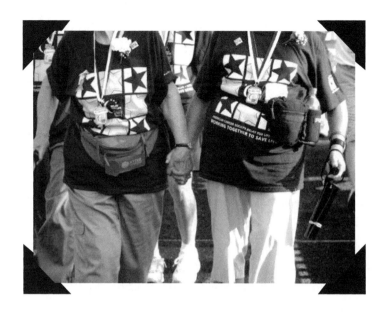

Walk with Me

Walking with a companion is an old-fashioned custom often lost in our modern era. There was once a time when walks home from school, from church, from a dance, or from a car to a front door were commonplace. Walking someone home was a way of offering protection and guidance–an opportunity to reflect on life and its experiences. I would like to invite you to come and take a walk with me. It's a perfect summer night with an illuminating aura surrounding us. How unusual to see so many walkers out tonight. As they pass by, I see smiles on their faces; but there is a certain sadness reflected in their eyes. Why is it that some of these pedestrians are pausing to embrace one another along the way? Some have walked loved ones "home," and there are tears streaming down their cheeks. These walking companions all seem to be wearing the same shirt that says "Relay for Life." I feel like I have just walked on sacred ground.

This past weekend I had many walking companions at the Renville County third annual Relay for Life in Minnesota co-chaired by my twin sister Meg and her husband. Over 1,000 hearts and hands connected for the cure as we all joined hands around the track swaying to the melody of "Love Can Build a Bridge." As the sun set on the 47 campsites, 6,100 luminaries were lit in honor of cancer survivors and in memory of those who have gone "home." At 4:30 a.m. I accompanied Meg to all the campsites to gather reflections for her closing ceremony. We asked our walking companions to describe the Relay in one word. The most interesting response came from a young man who said "juggernaut."

Juggernaut is a word used to describe a powerful, immovable force. What a great word to define this nationwide attempt to eradicate cancer. At 6:30 a.m., the 12 hour walkers gathered for the closing ceremony where hundreds of purple balloons were released to honor those who lost their lives on the cancer battlefield. The melody of "There You'll Be" from the movie *Pearl Harbor* lingers on in my mind. What a bittersweet celebration. Together we partied and ate, laughed and cried, played and prayed. Together we walked the full circle of life. Blessings to all as we walk with each other, beside each other, and... special blessings to those who have walked someone "home."

As we walk away from the Relay, please read the back of my survivor shirt. It says, ***"Dear Cancer, I win, YOU LOSE."***

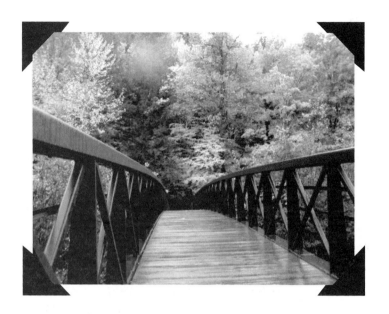

A Time for Everything

*E*very October it seems I find myself coming down with "nostalgiai-tis," which seems to cause an inflammation in my heart. The symptoms usually manifest themselves with a feeling of generalized restlessness, a bittersweet taste in my mouth, and a wistful yearning in my soul. What is it that I yearn for? I yearn for the past. I yearn for the days I would take my young sons on fall walks through the woods. I yearn for the days we would stuff scarecrows, pick pumpkins, frost Hal-loween cupcakes and cookies, and create the perfect costume for trick or treating. But there is one thing I yearn for more than anything...I yearn for my mom. She was only 52 when she was first diagnosed with uterine cancer...she was only 64 when she succumbed to colon cancer.

She died October 29, 1987. I was only 33. I still needed my mom, and my young sons still needed a grandmother. I am struggling to remember her voice, her touch, and, yes, even her appearance. I have brought out pictures, and I have brought out memories. I am trying to create a mental shrine. It's not about trick or treat anymore…it's about trinket or treasure. After my mom's death, my twin sister gave all of us siblings a framed prayer card along with this powerful message attached:

Trinket or Treasure

"A death has occurred and everything is changed by this event. We are painfully aware that life can never be the same again; that a relationship once rich was ended. But there is another way to look upon this truth. If life went on the same without the presence of the one who has died, we would only conclude that the life we have lost made no contribution, filled no space, meant nothing. The fact that this individual left behind a place that cannot be filled is a high tribute to them. Life can be the same after a trinket is lost, but never after a treasure."

~~Author Unknown

My mom was truly a treasure. My mom taught me how to "live" with cancer, not how to die with it. I was 42 when I was first diagnosed with ovarian cancer and 44 when I was diagnosed the second time. I yearned to have my mom come and hold me as I had held her in the end. She did come to me in a dream, and I will never forget her voice or the dress she wore. She said to me, "I am just so sorry." Mom, don't be sorry, for you taught me that there is a time for everything. You taught me how to be content with whatever I have. My mom raised me in a Christian home where we learned about life under the *son*.

"There is a time for everything and a season for every activity under heaven; a time to be born and a time to die, a time to plant and a time to uproot,

a time to kill and a time to heal, a time to tear down and a time to build,

a time to weep and a time to laugh, a time to mourn and a time to dance,

a time to scatter stones and a time to gather them,

a time to embrace and a time to refrain, a time to search and a time to give up,

a time to keep and a time to throw away, a time to tear and a time to mend,

a time to be silent and a time to speak, a time to love and a time to hate,

a time for war and a time for peace."

~~*Ecclesiastes 3: 18*

I miss you, Mom!

What a Wonderful World

*T*his morning I woke up to a room full of sunshine (I guess in the middle of winter that's a confession of sleeping in) with visions of a cup of coffee dancing through my head, and I thought to myself... what a wonderful world! I have many favorite hymns, but "What a Wonderful World" is my all time favorite song. As I sat with that cup of coffee, I listened to Eva Cassidy's rendition of "What a Wonderful World." For those of you who have never heard of her, Eva Cassidy was 33 when she was diagnosed with metastatic melanoma. Sadly, it was only after her death that her music was discovered throughout the nation. She had the immortal voice of an angel, and her CD "Songbird" is such a treasure.

I guess you could say that song has become my theme song, and I use it throughout my life to remind myself of the goodness in the world. Sometimes when we are in the middle of "stuff," it is easy to slip into a very unfashionable garment of sadness. Sometimes the first words out of our mouths in conversation are those of someone losing a job, going through a painful divorce, newly diagnosed with cancer, or battling a recurrence. Or perhaps the news is of someone with a child in trouble, someone awaiting test results; or worse yet, someone facing an imminent death unless they get their miracle. I charge myself as "guilty in the first degree." The above "stuff" is my "stuff."

I am glad that I have the kind of heart that I can render compassion for the pain of others, but it's like all things...we must find a balance. I am certain that this is something Dr. Matthews and the entire staff of MOA (Matthew's Oncology Associates) struggle with daily. My problem is that I have had so many people rally around me in my five year cancer experience that I want so badly to give back... sometimes to the detriment of my family and myself. How do I keep my life in check? I have learned to balance my emotional account. When I am feeling withdrawn, I know it's time for me to make another deposit. It is the reason I have learned the art of savoring moments. It is my way of re-depositing.

Today I remembered a deposit I had made two years ago. We were at a wedding in Chicago with some dear friends, all dressed up, and enjoying the ambiance and glitz of the city. As we returned to the hotel it was lightly snowing; and with a playful heart, I looked up the heavens and started singing my favorite song by Louis Armstrong:

I see trees of green, red roses too
I see them bloom for me and you
And I think to myself, what a wonderful world.

I see skies of blue and clouds of white
The bright blessed day, the dark sacred night
And I think to myself, what a wonderful world

The colors of the rainbow, so pretty in the sky
Are also on the faces of people going by
I see friends shakin' hands, saying "How do you do?"
They're really saying, "I love you."

I hear babies cryin', I watch them grow
They'll learn much more than I'll ever know
And I think to myself, what a wonderful world
Yes, I think to myself, what a wonderful world
Oh yeah

My New Year's resolution is to laugh louder, hug longer, listen more intently, and think to myself...what a wonderful world!

Magic Wand Therapy

Last night I walked into the living room with my usual basket of laundry and plopped myself on the floor to do my nightly task. Much to my surprise, there was actually something on TV worth watching. My husband Mark asked me if I had ever seen this movie before. Much to my delight, *Patch Adams* was on. I had indeed seen this powerful movie one other time while amidst the challenges of chemotherapy, and it made me weep for many reasons. Last night the movie took on a whole new dimension for me. For those of you who have never seen this classic, Robin Williams portrays a young, energetic, and eccentric pre-med student who became known to all as "Patch Adams." Patch Adams had a very nontraditional approach to medicine and was often ridiculed, disrespected, and criticized by his cohorts. He was indeed a colorful and playful person who practiced medicine outside of the box. He used humor, costumes, music, and whatever ingenuity it took to get his patients to eat, smile, stop throwing bedpans, laugh, love, and find peace in their final days. Patch Adams' beliefs were scrutinized; and in the end, he faced a review board to defend the one thing he wanted more than anything in life—he "just wanted to be a doctor." He gave a grand speech in his defense and defined a doctor. He said that a doctor is anyone who tries to improve the quality of someone's life by holding their hand, caring, and listening. His point was that if he was not allowed to practice medicine it would not stop him from being a doctor.

I could not help but think of Dr. Matthews throughout this movie because he not only practices medicine, but he is in the practice of being a doctor according to Patch Adams' definition. At one of my recent visits, Dr. Matthews shared a story with me of a woman who came in; and he had to give her a difficult diagnosis. He expressed his frustrations and sadness. Perhaps he thought or even said, "I just wish I could wave a magic wand and make it all disappear." The next day this woman appeared and delivered a gift to him...it was a magic wand. She told him it was a reminder for him that he can't always fix things for everyone. WOW, what an insightful and unselfish woman! At the end of my visit that day, Dr. Matthews waved his magic wand over me; we said a silent prayer together. Two weeks ago I again revisited Dr. Matthews and was delighted to see that I was in the magic wand room. I had great test results so; at my request, he once again shared this ritual with me. The beauty in this procedure is that it is free. You don't have to sign a Medicare disclosure for it. There is no prep, pre-medication, or fasting required. It requires no pre-authorization or a referral from your primary care physician. The magic wand therapy is pain free and non-invasive. It involves no scopes, needles, or claustrophobic machines.

What is so mystical about the magic wand therapy? It is a moment in time when you close your eyes, and you just know in your heart that even though it may not always be all right...it will always be okay! Thank you, Dr. Matthews for practicing medicine outside of the box. Thank you for practicing medicine holistically and with humanity. But most of all, thank you for your magic wand wishes!

Simply Simplify

*H*ave you noticed lately that people are crying out for a simpler life-style? The problem is that most of us don't know how to slow down our pace. Often times we carry around so many unnecessary burdens and responsibilities. We feel inadequate if we delegate duties, guilty when we say "NO," and overcome with selfishness if we even think about doing something for ourselves. Several months ago I was in an Amish store and saw some handcrafted items that read, "Simplify, Simplify, Simplify." What an appealing visual reminder in our cluttered and crazy lives. As I write for my column today, I am sitting in a simple space that I created just for me. It's a quiet place at the end of my upstairs hallway right by a window that has a view of a grand old tree that reaches up to the sky. There's a gentle breeze blowing through the window. I can hear the soothing melody of my wind chimes in the background, and my fountain is babbling peacefully. I am surrounded by my favorite things: my "HOPE" rock, my beautiful glass prism, a giant penny from Tim, a plant that I bought just for me, pictures that make me smile, and a big old basket of books.

Over the past two months, I have faced some health challenges. I was hospitalized for five days with a bowel obstruction, had CT scans, and sent to Madison for a P.E.T. scan. My physicians spoke of the high probability of a cancer recurrence or possible surgery if the symptoms did not resolve. I came home from the hospital weak and weary but immediately dove back into the "stuff" of life. Daily, I could feel myself sinking until I almost drowned. I was told by my physicians that I needed to take a leave of absence from work. I was forced to simplify my life. Unfortunately, there are no crash courses that teach you how to do this. In my self-taught studies on the art of simplification, I have learned that it all comes back to the basics of healing body, mind, and soul. Care of the body...well now that's an easy one to figure out. Basically, you just need to rest, eat healthy, and exercise. The challenge comes in implementing these foreign life-style changes. Care of the mind...this requires a little more ingenuity. For me, this is best achieved through reading, writing, and quiet time. But how do you heal your soul? In *Care of the Soul* by Thomas Moore we read, "Care of the soul isn't about doing, fixing, changing, adjusting, or making healthy; and, it isn't about some idea of perfection or even improvement. It doesn't look to the future for an ideal trouble-free existence. Rather it remains patiently in the present." To remain "patiently in the present" is a subject that I need frequent tutoring in. It requires me to take longer walks so that I can have prayerful discussions with my Teacher.

Cancer does have some privileges. I have been privileged to simplify my life for now. I have been given a grace period. I am embracing my life once again and truly enjoying long walks, chats with the neighbors, bird watching, the innocence of children, planting, painting, foot massages, sunsets, and Kemps Special Edition White Chocolate Raspberry Truffle ice cream. Recently a friend gave me a CD by Jim Brickman entitled "Simple Things." In his lyrics he says:

"HEY, time won't wait, life goes by,
Every day is a brand new sky,
Every tear comes to dry.
After all the clouds go by,
the simple things remain...
SIMPLE THINGS ARE FREE"

Forty-Five Minutes with God

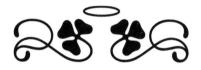

*H*ave you ever found yourself nodding your head vigorously while listening intently to someone telling a story? This gesture is our silent way of acknowledging and empathizing with someone's feelings, emotions, or experience. It is my hope that as my story unfolds you will all be sitting there with nodding heads. Several weeks ago, I went to our local hospital's walk-in clinic with a temp of 102 and a very painful sore throat. Seemed like a pretty "normal" and simple illness for a change...until I saw my chest x-ray. As I was in the x-ray department, my films were placed up on the viewing box for my uneducated viewing pleasure. I saw little white spots on my chest x-ray...a coincidental finding? Meanwhile an x-ray tech entered the room made a quick glance at my lungs, then at me, and stealthily removed the films. As she whispered something in another tech's ear, she proceeded to ask me, "Are you here alone today, Mary?" I was taken back to an exam room where another nurse appeared and again asked me, "Are you alone, Mary?" Indeed I was alone. I was alone with my self-diagnosis, my paralyzing thoughts, and with my God. During the next perpetual 45 minutes, I decided how I would tell my family of my recurrence. I updated my will and made arrangements for hospice. I made some mental notes of what I yet needed to tell my sons. I lamented for my grieving, lonely husband and chose a new partner for him. I consoled myself with having had six years since diagnosis. I felt confident that they would be able to keep me alive long enough to see my son get married in three months.

I reassured myself that my presence was of utmost importance and not appearance. I pondered on what my third wig should look like. I angrily reminded God that I had a new job at the Cancer Center that I love, a card line yet to launch, a book to write, and a son getting married. It just wasn't a convenient time to die. I had too much to do yet! At last the doctor came walking through the door; and as I prepared myself to hear those gut wrenching words for a third time, she said, "We can't seem to find anything Mary. I think it's all viral." How dare she tell me that I had a virus when I had just suffered, died, and buried myself alive? After a brief debate and deliberation, I finally accepted her un-dramatic diagnosis. My "little white spots" were my bronchi. Embarrassed and ashamed, I heralded my praises of thanksgiving and forgiveness.

Are you silently nodding? Have you ever been filled with fear and anxiety in precariously uncertain times? Did your mind create the worst possible scenario? What is the antidote to counteract such venomous thoughts? Confront your worst possible fears, say them out loud, share them with a loved one, write them down...learn to minimize what you have maximized. Pulitzer Prize winning author Anna

Quindlen said, "Consider the lilies of the field. Look at the fuzz on a baby's ear. Read in the backyard with the sun on your face. Learn to be happy. And think of life as a terminal illness; because if you do, you will live it with joy and passion as it ought to be lived." Today I asked my 20 year old son Luke, "What is the greatest lesson you have learned from cancer?" Without hesitation he responded, "How very precious life is."

Embrace the Mystery

A New York rescue worker buries his best friend after 9/11. "Why me?" he asks himself. Someone dies and donates an organ; the recipient asks, "Why me?" A war veteran stands in Soldier Field and asks himself, "Why me?" A plane crashes and the casualties outnumber the survivors. The survivors ask themselves, "Why me?" I was diagnosed with ovarian cancer and my twin sister asked herself, "Why me?" Why did I survive when others did not? Why is this happening to my child or my sibling instead of me? "Why me?" is a question that I asked myself last week after a phone call came from Dr. Matthews' office saying my PET/CT scan showed no cancer. The call came to me while at work at the Cancer Care Center on my seven year cancer-versary!

Why did I have to leave my work space to find a private corner to sob? "Why are you crying?" someone asked. "Aren't you happy?" "Of course I am happy and overwhelmed with gratitude." But why do I feel so sad and undeserving of this good news? Seven years ago when I was first diagnosed with cancer I asked, "Why me?" And today I find myself once again asking the same question; this time on the flip side. Why am I still alive while so many others who have faced my same diagnosis are not? Why am I doing so well when my friend has to suffer? Why am I statistically alive after facing this beast twice? I too am suffering...I am suffering from survivor guilt.

What is survivor guilt?

In a recent article, I read, "What Long-Term Survivors Don't Talk About" by Roberta Calhoun, ACSW, LICSW, she explains that not everyone experiences survivor guilt; it may vary in intensity, but it is a common experience. She further explains that many times caregivers experience survivor guilt for not being the one with the illness. Does survivor guilt have a function or a purpose? Calhoun goes on to say, "Survivor guilt may exist for a reason. It can help people find meaning and make sense out of their experiences. It may help survivors cope with the helplessness and powerlessness of being in a life threatening situation without the ability to protect or save others. More importantly, survivor guilt can co-exist with other responses, such as relief and gratitude, and may occasionally be prompted by them."

What purpose has survivor guilt served in my life?

I have always tried to find purpose to the events in my life, but it wasn't until this year's cancer-versary that I found purpose to the cancer in my life. It has been a year now since I have been working at the Cancer Care Center in Manitowoc. What greater purpose and meaning could I be given? In fact, that is where my S.G. (survivors' guilt) once again kicks in. How many people get to survive cancer twice and then get the opportunity to nurture and care for those who have been afflicted with the same disease? I am daily humbled and blessed with my encounters. The stories are enough to fill a book, but for now they fill my heart.

What can you do if you experience survivor guilt?

Robert Calhoun gives a list of seven ways to cope with survivor guilt. My personal favorite is, "Remind yourself that you are struggling to make sense of one of the greatest mysteries of the human race. Rather than explaining it away, try to embrace the mystery."

What did I do today to embrace the mystery?

I went out and planted a lot more perennials! Do I still suffer from S.G.? You bet I do. Every time I see a new patient walk through the doors of the Cancer Care Center I do. Am I still embracing the mystery? Yes, I am; and as long as I am alive, I will continue to do so.

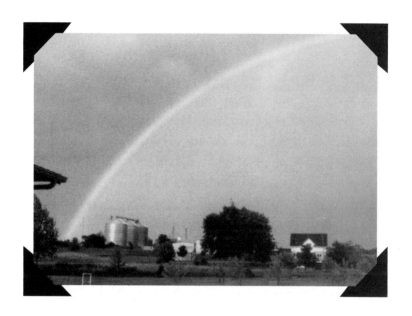

A Rainbow...Priceless!

Today, as I sat down at my computer ruminating over what I was going to write for my next "Hope Happenings" column, I received an amusing e-mail caricature of Noah's Ark. It portrayed all of the animals precariously peering over the edge of the ark observing a woodpecker busy at work pecking holes in their wooden vessel. At the front of the ark is Noah trying desperately to capture this formidable creature with a net. It made me laugh, so I printed it to put on my bulletin board in my office. My amusing cartoon soon became a visual simile. I couldn't help but think of the many diseases and circumstances that threaten to destroy our vessels.

Last week, I was privileged to have two days off in a row; so I decided to do something that I had been negligent in...helping others. On my way home from work, I stopped at the grocery store to make preparations for my cooking rampage. The following day was spent in my kitchen making comfort foods for four families who are having difficulty remaining afloat. Dirty pots and pans, messy kitchen, a whole day lost...PRICELESS! The next day was delivery day. Listening to the soul pain of others, sharing tears, playing cards with people who are visually and hearing impaired...PRICELESS! As I sat in the homes of my less fortunate friends and family, I almost felt an overwhelming sense of guilt and gratitude at the same time. They all have problems, diseases, and tenuous times; yet they continue to find joy in each and every day...PRICELESS! They all have things pecking holes in their lives threatening to sink their arks. The one thing that I heard in all of the conversations that priceless day was the love of their God, their family, and their friends.

What is the thing eating away at your life that is potentially destroying everything that you have worked so hard to build? Name it, claim it, say it...then IT may not seem so bad. Lastly, allow others to be a part of your vessel and to hold you up, for it is only then that the rainbow will be seen by all...PRICELESS!

Agatha Christie once said, "I have sometimes been wildly, despairingly, acutely miserable, racked with sorrows; but through it all, I still know quite certainly that just to be alive is a grand thing."

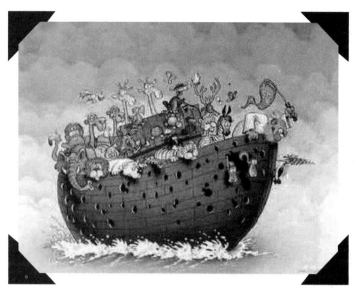

Everything I need to know about life, I learned from Noah's Ark...

One: Don't miss the boat.

Two: Remember that we are all in the same boat.

Three: Plan ahead. It wasn't raining when Noah built the Ark.

Four: Stay fit. When you're 600 years old,
someone may ask you to do something really big.

Five: Don't listen to critics;
just get on with the job that needs to be done.

Six: Build your future on high ground.

Seven: For safety's sake, travel in pairs.

Eight: Speed isn't always an advantage.
The snails were on board with the cheetahs.

Nine: When you're stressed, float a while.

Ten: Remember, the Ark was built by amateurs;
the Titanic by professionals!

Eleven: No matter the storm...
when you are with God there's always a rainbow waiting.

*Attributed and written by James Vuocolo (jim@soulbusiness.com).
Used with his permission.*

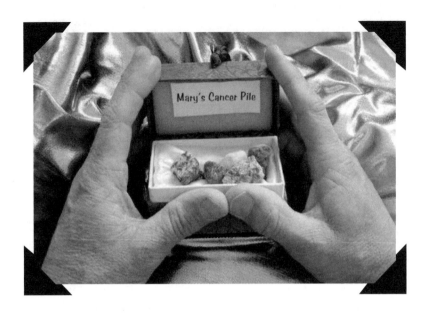

The Cancer Pile

*I*f perhaps you see a tear drop upon this story, it is my soul that is spilling over...a soul that has been tenderly and deeply touched. Allow me to share my husband's story.

Several weeks ago I spent two days up in Door County frolicking with my girlfriends. As any good wife does when she leaves home, I left a "Honey-do" list for my husband. I returned home on a hot Saturday afternoon somewhat surprised to see that Mark had chosen the project that was bottom on his list. Months ago he had a large load of gravel delivered into our yard with the intent of renting a Bobcat or skid loader to spread it out. Being a renowned procrastinator as well as being concerned about what this would cost, the gravel pile soon became a part of our yard. It was as if I didn't even see it anymore. In the heat of that day, I observed him digging into the pile, shoveling one load at a time on to his trailer, and spreading it out in the yard. Periodically I stood at my kitchen window and felt concerned yet quizzical. As he took numerous breaks to rest on our park bench, he sat with his arms folded upon his chest looking upward in a content and reflective manner. I marveled at his persistence and his stamina but questioned whether he would see it through to the end. Six hours later he completed his project.

That night as we sat outside together sipping on a glass of Door County wine, Mark said to me, "Do you know what that gravel pile was really all about?" He shared with me that he contemplated quitting and renting a skid loader so that he "wouldn't kill himself." He said that he knew he needed to set himself a goal and that's when he "started his journey." He called his gravel pile "Mary's cancer pile." With this new found goal in mind, he decided to "pick at it little by little." He "wasn't going to quit until he got it done." He reflected, "It was hard work! Many times I had to stop and rest because I was so tired. My heart was pounding so fast. I needed to just catch my breath and then go back at it. That's kind of the way Mary's treatments went. Every treatment was another little battle that she had to keep doing. When it got down to the very end, I thought, well I just have a small pile left. Now I'm really going to go at it...I'm going to give it my all. But I had to stop one more time until my body was rested again. I finally got the job done."

Somehow this ominous pile of dirt had become a curative transfiguration of healing. In a book by Dr. Robert Hopcke, he says, "Searching for meaning to events on a daily basis will add spark to your life because it's a creative act. If you cultivate a contemplative attitude, a way of consistently looking for the significance of even chance events, you'll begin to see the meaning." In a pile of gravel, my husband not only found meaning; he felt my pain.

There is one final thing that I must now do. I need to go outside and place some of those precious gems in a box to give to Mark. Perhaps it will always be a reminder for him to search for meaning underneath the pile.

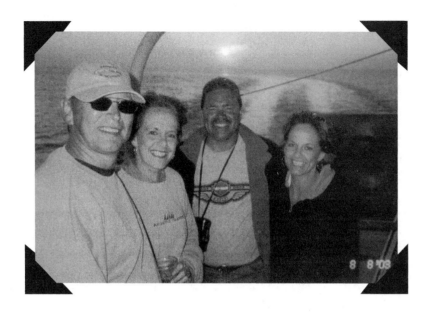

8 8 '03

Applauding the Ordinary

When was the last time you put your hands together extolling praise or celebration? Perhaps it was at a birthday or retirement party, upon the completion of a race, or when that special someone graduated with honors. Was it when you witnessed a toddler taking their first steps? Or was it that magical moment in time when two young lovers are declared husband and wife? Perhaps it was as you sat in church with your hands folded and your head bowed giving glory, laud, and honor to our Heavenly Father.

Allow me to set the background for my ordinary, laudatory moment. Just this past week, my husband and I along with my twin sister and her husband vacationed together. We camped for three glorious days along the captivating shores of Lake Superior in Bayfield, Wisconsin. We visited the home of an artist, and we strolled the reflective trails that keep her energized and fueled in creativity. We picked stones on the beach and swam in the transparent waters of the Chequamegon Bay. We encountered a set of identical male twins and mirrored tales of double trouble and the phenomena of twinship. We shopped to the best of our ability, trying earnestly to misplace our husbands. We ate a lot and slept too little. We enjoyed fine wine, s'mores, glowing bonfires, and a Tic tournament (a new card game that challenged us to actually think periodically). We spent one day exploring Madeline Island learning of the history of the Apostle Islands from a colorful and seasoned islander. We incredulously marveled at the abounding beauty of God's exterior decorating. The air was crisper, the stars were brighter, and I don't think I have ever seen a fuller moon...and then one day the sun set.

On that day, we boarded a ferry for a three hour tour...yes, a three hour tour. We voyaged to a few islands receiving yet another history lesson along the way. We viewed lighthouses and learned about life as a lighthouse keeper. We were awe-struck by the mystical formations of the caves...and then we were bored. We begged Mark to let us crack open our bottle of wine that was originally reserved for a sunset toast. Gratefully, he did not cave in to our pleas. In anticipation of this ordinary event, everyone searched for the best seat in the house, loaded their cameras with fresh film, and focused their binoculars to get a closer look. As the sun slowly reached the horizon irradiating a showcase of color on Lake Superior, we finally cracked open our wine. We toasted to life, and then it happened. This daily event turned into something laudable as everyone on the upper deck put their hands together and applauded the sunset. Meg and I musingly questioned, "What's up with that?" We both agreed that it was not about celebrating this daily occurrence or its splendor. What people were really applauding was that they took the time to see it as though it was for the first time.

What a wonderful reminder of life's essentials: food, water, shelter, and recreation! Recreation is a vital element in our re-creation. It gives us the opportunity to re-create our relationships away from the daily distractions of life. It gets us back in touch with what's important in life and sharpens our priority skills. It re-creates our values making them invaluable. Recreation is a refresher course in laughter, relaxation, and play. It stimulates our senses and rejuvenates our spirit. It is mind-altering therapy that puts us in slow motion. Recreation re-creates our focus on the present. It is turning the ordinary into the mementos. May your life be full of applaudable sunsets.

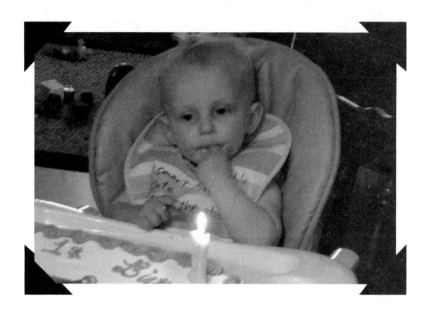

Dip into Life

Several months ago I had the honor of meeting a young child named Dakota. I was getting my hair "rejuvenated" (what a blessing to have hair) when this little person came walking in. To be honest, I did not know if he was a he...or if he was a she. This child hopped up into the chair; and as locks of hair fell to the floor, it soon became apparent that HE was getting HIS first big boy first grade haircut! He looked fearful; and yet with each snip of the scissors, he seemed to sit higher in the chair. He looked precariously into the mirror as his younger siblings and parents looked on. He squirmed feverishly as most children do when feeling un-environmentally safe. Perhaps his feeling of uncertainty came from seeing me sitting under the dryer looking like

I was preparing for Halloween in mid-August. With each snip of the scissors, Dakota became a little more wary especially when the stylist started to cut around his ears. It was with great concern that he gently spoke up, "Don't cut my ear off!" The stylist tenderly replied, "I haven't lost one yet today." As I listened to his concerns, I added, "Dakota, you are going to need those ears for first grade." And he added, "And my nose to smell...and my *fingers* to taste." At that point Dakota not only had a big boy haircut, but he had a big life message! As he hopped out of the chair, his hairdresser said, "I bet you are going to be able to run a lot quicker now." He retorted, "I will be able to run away from the girls."

Dakota taught me a lot in his brief booster seat rhetoric with a dinosaur cape draped around his neck. He was a little person with a big life. For a brief moment in time, I was so jealous of him; and I longed to be six years old again tasting the simplicity of life with my fingers. When do we stop being childish and get so grownupish? What happens to us as adults that we become so conservative in our thoughts, so un-inquisitive, so regimented, and so very complicated? What happens to our senses that we can no longer make sense of our lives? Fear seems to consume all of our senses. We fear failure; and yet, we fear the challenges that come with success. It blinds us! We fear hearing what others might say about us if we dare to step outside of the box. It deafens us! We think that life is unfair and even stinks at times. We stop smelling the roses! We search for ways to become numb so that we can stop feeling. We fear life, and we fear death. We fear the bitter and forget to taste the sweet.

That day back in the salon, not only was my color rejuvenated, but so was the spirit of the child locked up inside of me. Dakota, thank you for reminding me to not be so grownup-ISH!! Thank you for teaching me how to dip into life and taste with my *fingers*.

Mmm, Mmm, Mmm...Life is so sweet!

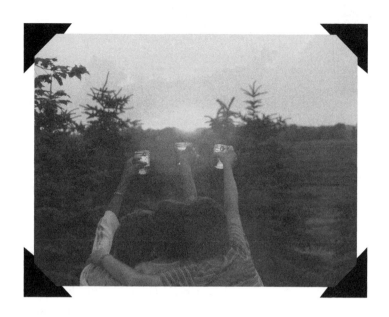

Love...
a Many Splendored Thing

It is the day after Valentine's Day; and as I sit at my keyboard, my heart is reverberating the sweet sentiments of the past two days. It all started on Friday night when I attended a Jim Brickman concert with two loving cherubs for a girls' night out. We are three kindred spirits whose lives have been soldered together. One of our mutual physicians dubbed us "The Fork Ladies" after seeing a framed photograph of the three of us with a glass of wine in one hand and a fork in the other. We were toasting life but saving our forks for we know that the best is yet to come. We all have fork earrings and an angel necklace that are mandatory apparel when we gather monthly for our "Fork Ladies" night out. We take pictures at each gathering and have a "Fork Ladies" photo album. Sometimes we cry together, but mostly we laugh. We always treasure and savor our times together finding some reason to celebrate. You see the alloy that has united the three of us as tines on a fork is cancer.

Together we have shared remissions and recurrences, good test results and bad. We have traveled with each other to doctor appointments and held bedside vigils during hospitalizations. We have decorated hospital rooms and IV poles with the abundance of a Thanksgiving Day feast. We philosophize together, give foot and hand massages, watch movies, discuss books and music, pick raspberries, have bonfires, and eat s'mores. We talk about kids, husbands, life, love, and even death. We have attended sessions on planning your own funeral, shared discussions on advance directives and cremation. We attend National Cancer Survivors Day together, and we walk the survivor lap hand in hand at Relay for Life. We pray for each other, we pick each other up when one falls down, and we restore each other's hope when one is downcast. I cannot imagine my life with a missing prong! During our Valentine's concert, Jim Brickman talked about the many different kinds of love people have for each other. It was indeed a special moment when we all embraced each other's hands and on the count of three were urged to kiss the person next to us. Tears welled up in my eyes and a sob came to my throat as I realized that what we have is a gift from God...we have an "agape love."

Last night I made a date with my husband of 29 years for Valentine's Day. We got all dressed up for dinner and enjoyed the ambiance of a very special night out on the town. I could not stop smiling because I felt so special; I felt so loved. He gave me a beautiful card that iterates what love is all about. "We surely know our love survives through everything we face. This cherished bond we've shared so long could never be replaced. That's why I've never minded—as many people do—growing slowly older, for I'm growing old with you." We came home that evening, put some music on, and danced on our newly refurbished kitchen floor. As we danced, I reflected on the unconditional love of this man who loved me though cancer twice. He loved me when I was bald, sick, and scared. Tears welled up in my eyes and a sob came to my throat again as I realized that what we have is a gift from God...we have an "agape love."

There have been many studies done on love that include the exploration into the different types of love and the various ways men and women express love. For those of you not familiar with the term "agape love," it is the unselfish love of one person for another likened to the love of God for mankind. Agape love is a self-sacrificing love, an altruistic love that is experienced by people willing to do things for another person with no expectations in return. It is an unselfish and unconditional kind of love for each other. It is a kind of love that says, "I will be here for you...no matter what!"

During this time of love and romance, for all of you who may be feeling sad or lonely because you do not have that "romantic" kind of love in your life, I urge you to look around. I am certain that you have an agape kind of love in your life. Perhaps you did not get a dozen red roses on Valentine's Day; but, agape love has a far sweeter fragrance for it is precious, beloved, and revered. It is the essence and sustenance of life and true love!

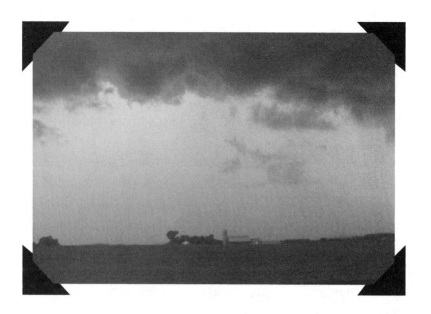

Tornado Slices Through Countryside

"Tornado Slices Through Countryside." These were recently the headlines of our little local newspaper with a subtitle that read, "We were damned scared!" On July 13 as I was about to depart to Sheboygan for a three month visit with Dr. Matthews, the skies suddenly grew solemn and eerie. I called Denise to cancel my appointment and then decided to turn the TV on. A tornado had touched down in Clarks Mills and was headed between JJ and 151...THAT'S ME I surmised in a frenzy! How can this be happening? There were no sirens or warnings, and now I am about to be caught up in a funnel cloud in five minutes! I quickly grabbed the portable phone, my personal phone directory, and scrambled to my old farmhouse basement. It was there that

I found refuge along with some arachnids and arthropods. I hastily dialed up my husband praying that he would answer his cell phone. His voice never sounded sweeter..."Where is the best place to go? Should I be doing anything else? Stay on the line with me!" I pleaded. Fourteen and a half minutes later I let him hang up as we only had high winds and hail. I thanked God for the roof that was still over my head and even the little creatures within. News reports were coming in citing that people were wandering around in shock. Our rural neighbors had lost a home, barns were down, and local enforcement was sent out to assess the damage. It was described as "a complete devastation", but everyone survived. In the aftermath of the storm, the clean up began. Disaster relief funds had been established, and people were trying to resume some sense of normalcy. They mourned their losses, knowing in their hearts that life would never be the same again.

Cancer is so much like a tornado that slices through our lives. Without any warning signs or sirens going off, the diagnosis abruptly touches down and swoops you up in a funnel cloud where you are caught spinning and spinning. The fear of death is surreal with scattered, frenzied thoughts flying through the air like broken pieces of our lives. What am I going to tell my loved ones? How will my kids survive without me? I'll never get to see that graduation, that prom, that wedding day, that trip, etc. Who is going to hold my kids in their arms, my first grandchild, my spouse? I was devastated and in shock. And, yes, I was "damned scared" when the tornado touched down twice in my life. But then the storm dissipates. In the aftermath, you assess the damage: chemo brain, neuropathy, no hair, no eyelashes, no eyebrows, no ovaries, no uterus, no energy, no appetite, no life... no normalcy. BUT PRAISE BE TO GOD...I was saved! Recovering from a disaster is never an easy task. But with the help of God, family, friends, professionals, and even strangers...all things are possible. The next time you see someone devastated by the storms of life, assess the damage; and perhaps, in some small way, you can be a special part of their disaster relief fund.

In Mark 10:26-27 the disciples asked Jesus,
"Who then can be saved?"
Jesus looked at them and said,
"With man this is impossible, but not with God;
All things are possible with God."

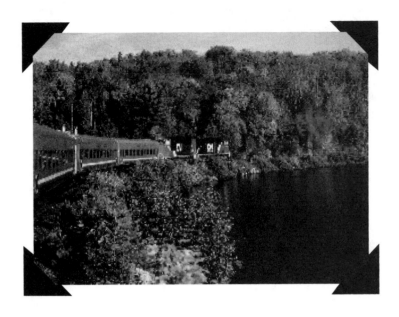

Life's Canyons

Last week my husband and I escaped for a few days on a fall excursion to the exquisite shores of Lake Michigan, Lake Superior, and Lake Huron. It was a sensuous sanctuary of color and crisp lake breezes. Horns blared as majestic vessels navigated through the channels of the Sault Ste. Marie locks. Our palates were aroused with morsels of fresh lake fish and the finesse of fine wine. We reveled in a Canadian sunset on Lake Huron with the impressive international bridge as a backdrop. But the highlight of our explorations was our one day train tour to the Agawa Canyon. Aboard the Algoma Central railway, we wound our way through the heart of 22,000 square miles of recreational wilderness. We marveled at the visionary pallet of blaze red, orange, and green. Once arriving in the lush valley, we ventured on the trails which led us to serene waterfalls and sites for some great Kodak moments. Amongst nature we sat and lunched on train-made Minestrone soup and sandwiches, thanking God for respite time.

Before re-boarding the train, I quizzically asked my husband, "How are we going to get back out of the canyon?" You don't just make a u-turn in a canyon or put a train in reverse. The query was revealed when we observed the engineers disengage the engine placing it in the rear, and the caboose was orchestrated to the front to conduct the trip home. One question remained, would we be looking backwards in our seats all the way home? The train whistle resounded against the canyon walls summoning us "All Aboard!" We were fascinated as we returned to our seats to find that all of the seats had been rotated around. We were facing ahead to begin our journey home.

Have you ever been caught in a deep narrow valley with sides so high that you cannot foresee a way out? Has depression, an addiction, disease, disability, a job loss, or a life-altering situation left you feeling hopeless? Do you find yourself sitting backwards in the seat of life always looking at the caboose? Perhaps you need to swivel your chair around and face forward. If we spend all of our lives looking back, we may fail to see the beauty that lies ahead. We are the conductors of our lives! We can choose to look back, or we can choose to focus our attention on what lies in front of us. With God as our engineer and the help of family, friends, and trained professionals, we *can* pull ourselves out of the canyons in life. As the chugging of the train echoes in my mind, I can't help but think of a wonderful tale of self-strength written by Watty Piper...*The Little Engine That Could.* May his famous rallying mantra resonate in the hearts and souls of all those who may perceive that they are stuck in a canyon.

"I THINK I CAN...I THINK I CAN...I THINK I CAN!"

Believe in the Magic

*H*ave you ever had an event occur in your life that you just can't seem to forget...a happening that makes you wonder, "What was that really all about?" Has someone's life ever touched yours for a brief moment in time, yet their face and their narrative linger on long after the encounter?

Last week I attended the annual Holiday Social at the Cancer Care Center where I work. The chemo bay was full of the hope of Christmas as cancer survivors gathered with friends and family to celebrate life. I was absorbed in wonderment as I stood back observing the gaiety among so many who are physically broken yet spiritually whole. It was at that time that I noticed a young man standing alone in the doorway. I am ashamed to say that initially I hesitated to approach him as his face was unfamiliar and his appearance was tattered and tousled. As he lingered in the doorway scanning the room, there was something that drew me to him. I approached this stranger uncertain if I was going to invite him in or encourage him to leave, that is, until I looked into his eyes and saw a lost soul. I asked him if he was looking for a friend or family member to which he responded, "No." He said that he "wasn't sure why" he was there; that someone had "opened the door and invited him in." I asked him if he was hungry, and he said that he was. I invited him in. He put some food on a plate, sat down on a chair, and proceeded to study the crowd as I studied him. I finally went and sat next to him and inquired if cancer had affected his life in some way? He gave a sketchy encounter of his mother dying at the age of 61... "She had tumors. I think colon cancer." I introduced myself and learned that his name was Tim. In the next ten minutes, Tim shared his sorrows, his dreams, his life. Since the passing of both parents, it saddened Tim that his seven siblings never gathered anymore. "All they do is quarrel," he said. He further explained that his parents were the ones who kept it all together. He never married because he wasn't good at relationships. "I have always been kind of a grouch." Tim shared that he was laid off from his job, but he had a dream to save up enough money to tour the U.S. on his bike. He told me that he has problems with his lower legs being numb and painful. And then Tim made eye contact and said, "I don't know why I am telling you all of this. I have never told anyone these things before." He asked me why everyone in the room seemed so happy. My heart was deeply moved when Tim professed, "I think the reason I am here tonight is because I need to be around positive people. And you know what else? Today is my birthday!" It was apparent to me that his past birthdays were uneventful as he was uncertain how old he was. "Forty-one or forty-two...born in 1961." I told Tim that I hated to burst his bubble, but he was forty-three years old. I ran and got some cake and balloons and gathered a group to sing "Happy Birthday" to Tim. As he proudly stood, tears filled his eyes and silence fell over the entire room. It was as though he was hearing this birthday ballad for the first time in his life. When he sat down, he stared at his impromptu cake as though it was the greatest gift anyone had ever given him...perhaps it was. Before departing I made sure that Tim knew that there were community resources available if he needed food or shelter and invited him to join us again next year.

As I walked outside, the first snowfall of winter was gently falling to the ground. I felt like something so magical had happened...I had met "Tiny Tim!" I not only believe in the magic; but first and foremost, I believe in the Magi. When you believe...you *will* receive. God opened a door that night, and what a privilege it was to be His greeter. I believe God has made me mindful of the greatest gift we can give others—the gift of our presence. I believe that God has made me mindful of the greatest gift we can receive—the gift of His son.

"Keep on loving each other as brothers. Do not
forget to entertain strangers, for by so doing some
people have entertained angels without knowing it."
~Hebrews 13:1-3

May you believe in the magic. May you believe in the miracle of Jesus.

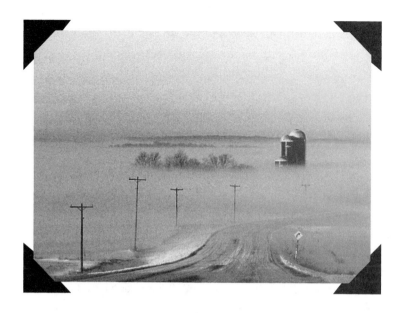

Life Altering Events

~~*by Mark Matthias*

It has been almost a year since my family surprised me with a digital camera for Christmas. I work for the farming community so it takes me to the countryside and into the back roads. There were many occasions that I wished I would have had a camera. My wish had finally come true.

Learning to use a digital camera is one thing, but so much of taking a great picture is just being at the right place at the right time. So many times it's when the sunlight is peeking through a cloud or the fog is just starting to lift or some form of wildlife is showing its face. So many times a "would be" picture presented itself, but I didn't have my camera. Now my camera goes with me every day.

It's been almost ten years since Mary's diagnosis of cancer. It was a day I wish I could forget, but I know I won't. I was doing some soil sampling that day, which means I am out of my truck for hours at a time with no communication. I had a cell phone, but it wasn't the nice compact and portable ones they have now. I don't think there was much of a voice message service either. I do remember that day there was a phone number that showed up on my screen, but I didn't recognize it. I would come to find out that it was Mary trying to contact me. Well, the rest is history...I was absolutely at the wrong place at the wrong time.

I've heard it said that you should not let cancer become your friend. There really aren't any benefits of having cancer. However, it definitely gives you a whole new framework on how you live your life. I truly believe it has had an effect on so many life decisions—decisions that would probably have been different if cancer had not occurred.

As Mary went through her treatments, she always set new goals. The first I remember so well. She wanted to see the Grand Canyon. Through the generosity of her co-workers, they made it happen. I remember not only the awesome display of God's artwork but the sight of Mary hugging her twin sister and the quiet whispering to each other "we did it" (no digital camera here—but that image will be in my mind forever).

It has been God's will that Mary has been able to reach all of her goals. She has seen her sons graduate from high school, witnessed their getting married to some very wonderful and beautiful ladies, having the opportunity to watch them grow as they chose their careers. But the most awesome event of all is seeing her hold her first grandchild. Yes, Leah Rose was born October 27, 2005. It is so humbling to hold the beginning of another generation of your own flesh and blood in your hands.

Cancer is not our friend, but I can't help but wonder if the events in our lives would not have had the humbling, heartfelt meaning that they do now? Would our sons have chosen different careers? Ryan is in the medical field as a Radiography Technologist in the cardiac cath/special procedures lab where he met his wife while going through school. Luke will soon be graduating from UW Oshkosh as a teacher...a decision he made because he wanted to make a difference in the lives of young people and the world. Would the meaning of this new grandbaby not be quite as grand? Would our lives be more tuned into materialistic things? These are all questions that don't have a complete answer, but I do believe that life-altering events render themselves to life-altering decisions.

So, I'll enjoy my digital camera this Christmas Season, saving memories and taking lots of images of grandbabies. Lots and lots of images...I can get over 125 on one disc!

Have a Blessed Christmas and a Happy New Year.

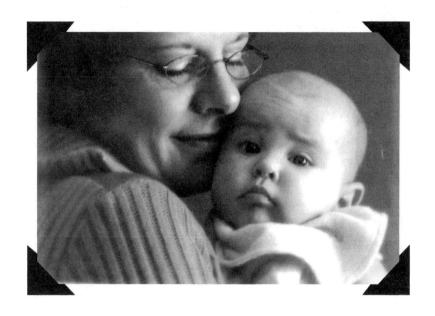

Am I Crazed?

It all started about four months ago. I began to notice every female child on earth as though this species was nonexistent prior to this time. Then there is this strong magnetic force that keeps sucking me into every baby section of any store I walk into (even the grocery store lures me to places I have not been in 27 years). I aimlessly wonder around...feeling, smelling, squeaking, reading, and playing. I catch myself watching the computer for photos and listening to babbling messages on my answering machine over and over and over. But the most disturbing of all these anomalies is that I have become a "closet bib sniffer"! I am preoccupied, obsessed, and have been accused of being crazed. Is there a support group for people like me? What hexes me to behave in such a bizarre manner? Her name is Leah Rose, and I have entered the bewitching phenomena of GRAND-parenting.

In the early days A.G. (after grandchildren), I walked around thinking that I must look different–surely someone will notice the aura around me. I remember going to the grocery store with my new brag book in hand announcing to Gramps that I probably would not be returning for several hours, depending on who I all ran into. At times when I am in a hurry to get in and out, I have been known to dodge conversations. But on this particular Saturday afternoon, I loitered, patrolling each aisle for a friend or even a simple acquaintance so that I could reveal "the most beautiful child in the world." I was in my final moments of desperation at the check-out counter when it behooved me to strike up a conversation with the bagger, after all my son attended high school with her six years ago. She so graciously pretended to be interested.

Then there was the day that I had a colonoscopy. I told Dr. Shariff that I would not allow him to sedate me until he looked at my pictures. In order to appease me and not run behind schedule, he took a few minutes to dote on my grandbaby.

In January we went to Orlando and spent a day at Epcot. I found myself having conversations with total strangers about their babies and observing every grandparent's interaction with their grandchild. I dreamed of one day seeing Disney through the eyes of Leah.

Just recently I subscribed to a magazine called "GRAND." It is filled with grand stories, grand advice, grand ideas, grand pictures, and info on grand trips to take with your grandchildren. Today I was online searching for books to teach me the repertoire of skills that I will need to possess if I am to be successful in this grand new role.

Every two to three weeks, we pack our bags for an overnight visit so that we can bond with this new little creature. It is simply euphoric to see her sweetly sleeping in the stillness of the night and to hear her babbling with delight in the newness of the day. At naptime I swaddle her in my arms escaping to a quiet place. There we sit and rock. I feel her tiny heart resounding against mine. I feel the synchronized rhythm of her breathing. I study her growing eyelashes, her rosebud nose, her lips that so resemble her mother's, her delicate fingers clasped around mine. There I sit and weep.

Why do I weep? My tears are not that of a crazed woman. My tears come from a soul that is simply inundating with gratitude. In May I will celebrate my ten year, two time ovarian "Cancerversary." At my first visit to Dr. Matthews' office, I also wept. My tears came from a tremulous body, a paralyzed mind, and a heart that was broken. I told Dr. Matthews that one day I wanted to become a Grandma; when in reality, I was thinking I would never see my sons graduate from high school. Leah Rose is a gift of grandness that goes beyond anything I ever asked for or dared to dream of.

Someone asked me the other day if I was going to be this crazed when my second grandchild arrives. My response was, "I certainly plan on it!" Perhaps I am a bit crazed, although I prefer to think of it as being passionate about my new purpose in life. The Zen of grand-parenting has taken me to a state of "no-mind." It has taught me the skill of being deliberately present in silence. Elisabeth Kubler-Ross once said, "Learn to get in touch with the silence within yourself and learn that everything in life has purpose. There are no mistakes, no coincidences; all events are blessings given to us to learn from." Thank you, Leah Rose, from you I have learned the grandness of stillness.

~~Oma Mary

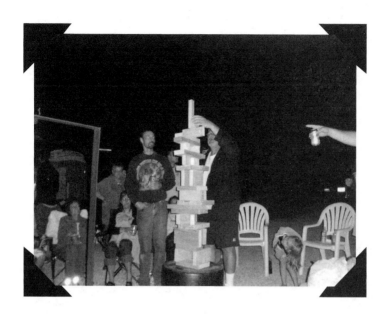

Jenga®...A Game of Life

I think my son, the new teacher, has rejuvenated in me a sense of curiosity about history and happenings. He has taught me that as an adult it is still okay to question the five W's...who, what, when, where, and why. Although I must admit at times I ask, "Who really cares? Well, who really cares about Jenga ®? Well I didn't care until recently, and then I asked the questions. Here are the facts:

Jenga ® was invented in the early 1970s by Leslie Scott, a British citizen who spent some teen years living in Africa. To name her game, she coined the term Jenga ®, a Swahili word meaning "to build." The wood blocks for the game began as alder trees, considered weeds and of little value. More recently, it has been discovered that alder is an important source of hardwood, making it useful as a strong building material.

In August my family came together for our second annual Riesterer Rally. We gathered as siblings and spouses, welcoming our children and grandchildren. We are just a simple family coming together on a yearly basis trying to keep our family roots alive without our parents to hold us together anymore. We enjoy each other's company, we renew our historical roots and values, we catch up on one another's lives, we meet new family members, we create new memories, and we reminisce about the old. The highlight of that year's event was campfire Jenga ® introduced by my brother Leo. We were there *"to build."* On that special Saturday night as the moon lit up the sky, we once again gathered full circle around the bonfire. I saw my brother dump a plastic tote of varying sizes of pre-cut building blocks around the fire. It was his invitation for young and old to partake in "Campfire Jenga ®." We were all told that the importance of the game was to build a solid foundation. Our goal as a family was to build the highest tower without letting it fall. We had spotters on board to protect people from falling blocks. We celebrated strategic planning, and we were supportive of decisions that were made unwisely. It was all in fun...it was all about building.

Our building was really all about bonding. As a family, we have won the game of Jenga ®. We already have plans to gather and build again for many years to come. Our foundation is made of strong building material...faith, family, and friends.

How to Win the Game

- You are a winner when you are weak...let others reinforce you.
- You are a winner when you are falling...let others catch you.
- You are a winner when you have fallen...let others build you up.

- You are a winner when you have learned the game plan... build a solid foundation.

"We're conditioned to think that our lives revolve around great moments. But great moments often catch us unaware—beautifully wrapped in what others may consider a small one."

~~Pastor Timothy Burt

"A Sorrow Shared Is Half the Sorrow. A Joy Shared Is Twice the Joy!"

"A Swedish Proverb"

When Tim told me the quote for the next newsletter, I couldn't help but ponder on the joy that has come back to me twofold in my work at the Cancer Care Center in Manitowoc. It is there in the heart of the chemo bay that we commiserate together, yet it is there that we find daily celebrations. We don our cheerleading uniforms and shake our pom-poms when we hear such things as stable, remission, negative findings, significant response, within the normal range, treatment completed. There is no such thing as ordinary in our repertoire of words. Every event becomes an extraordinary happening. We blow up balloons, order cake, and croon when someone grows old. We gather for bell ringing ceremonies upon completion of chemo or radiation.

We rejoice over vacations, anniversaries, graduations, grandbabies, and goals that have been reached. It is so easy to become a good cheer-leader. There are instructors, coaches, and camps to teach you how to become the best; but what about the sorrow-leaders? How do we become skilled? Who are our teachers? How do we gain confidence in our routines?

As a nurse, I was recently challenged at being a sorrow-leader; and I prayed that God would show me how. Penny has been a very special teacher to all of us. She has faced numerous adversities, always appears to be so upbeat, and always finds the courage to dive in... again and again. On this particular day, Penny was very discouraged with news of test results; her treatment plan was being altered...she had another bend in the road. She was so down that day, as was I. I remember going into the restroom trying to regroup. I was feeling so helpless not knowing what to say...not knowing what to do. A part of me, pathetically, wanted to avoid Penny and John. Then I looked into the mirror and instantly knew what I needed to do. I went out into the chemo bay; and without a word, I knelt at Penny's chair. I took the necklace off that I had worn that day and placed it around Penny's neck. It was a necklace that had a pink studded ring around it that bore the word "Hope." I told her that I was putting *hope* around her neck... it was used *hope,* and I hoped that she did not mind. I called Penny to ask her permission to share this story. She agreed and these were her words, "That moment was sacred to me. I was so very touched that someone would take something off their neck and place it around mine. The fact that it *was* "used" only made it more special to me." Penny told me that she has only taken the necklace off once and that was to have her hair colored. Another reason to celebrate...she had hair. Penny, thank you for allowing me to share our story. It was an in-timate moment in my life that will be forever embedded in my heart.

Charles Dickens once wrote, "It was the best of times, it was the worst of times." Thank you, Penny, and so many others who have taught me that simple moments are stellar moments. Those are the moments that humble me daily...they truly are "Hope Happenings."

Addendum: *We celebrated Penny's "life" on Dec. 20, 2008 after her earthly departure. "May the Lord Bless You and Keep You." Kelly, Kari, and Lauren you were everything... "In Your Mother's Eyes." Just to let you know the pink studded "Hope" necklace now lies around the neck of and in the heart of Julie, Penny's loving sister who embraced her and her dying wishes until the end! Julie, may you always cherish those last shopping days together for the best Christmas gifts ever, those future wedding gifts that the girls would treasure forever, and those baby shower gifts that Penny chose for the grandchildren she would never see! God bless all care-givers! There is no medication strong enough to take away your pain. There is no treatment to cure your broken hearts.*

You Gotta Have TUDE

What is the first thing you do when you awaken in the morning? Do you hit the snooze button for just a few more winks of shut-eye? Are you one of those who have to have a cup of coffee before you can function? Do you lie in bed and listen to the morning news, plan your day, meditate, or pray? Or are you one of those ambitious people who hop on the treadmill, head out the door for a walk, or perhaps a workout at the fitness center? One thing is certain; we are all creatures of individual habits. But there is one thing that we ALL do every day, some consciously and others unconsciously. We all choose the apparel that we are going to don. When you go to your closet, don't forget to choose the most essential accessory of the day...attitude.

Last week I happened to be off on an incredibly warm, sunny spring day. I was running errands when I began to notice some very peculiar events. My curiosity was aroused. Why did that woman let me ahead of her in the check-out? Why are so many strangers smiling at me? Why did that man motion for me to go ahead of him when we were gazing at the same parking spot? Why does everyone seem to be engaged in lazy, lingering conversations? The whole world was stunningly accessorized with joy-filled and gracious attitudes. That night as I shared my observations with my husband, he commented, "And what will happen when it's 95 degrees out?"

Several years ago when I was cancering for the second time, someone gave me a vital accessory. I was given a t-shirt that professed these words:

"At-ti-tude \ n: you gotta have 'tude
If you're gonna take a lickin'
And keep on kickin'."

Indeed we all do need to have 'tude. 'Tude is what you need to put on the first thing every morning. 'Tude is the stuff that will see you through those days when the sun isn't shining and there are dark clouds overhead. 'Tude is what you will need to see your way through life's storms.

'Tude is available to everyone...you just have to know where to find it.

*'**Tude** is found in gratitude.*
In M. J. Ryan's book *"Attitudes of Gratitude"* it is written:
"And the greatest thing is that as we experience the mental sunshine of gratitude, we begin to glow with sunshine ourselves. Suddenly not only is the world brighter, but we are too. Soon we notice that our lives are full of people who want to be around us because we exude peacefulness, happiness, and joy."

When you find *'tude,* make sure to wear it everyday. It will compliment you! It will become the most essential part of your daily ensemble.

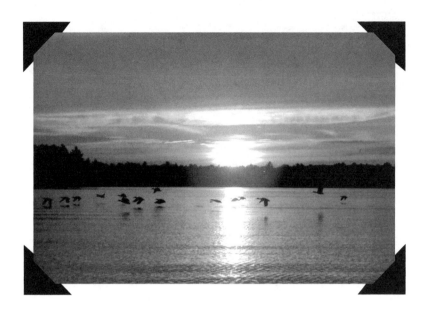

I'm Movin' On

It is a beautiful day outside...72 degrees; and truthfully, there is not a single cloud in the bluest of skies. It is one of those days where you thank God for HIS artistry, acoustics, and aromas. It is truly a perfect day. My old quilt and sheets are gently flapping in the breeze much like a butterfly in flight. In the background there is the hum of lawn mowers, tractors, and my husband working on outdoor projects. It's an easy day...my favorite kind. Then why is it that I am feeling so melancholy? Perhaps it is because I am mourning the loss of those 35 year old pine trees that had to go down this year. And that grand old Basswood that threatened to be on our roof is recently gone too. And now it is time to empty pots, cut back perennials, chop corn, mow the lawn one last time, and prepare the house for winter. And I wonder,

"Is anyone hanging Christmas lights?" Meanwhile my mind is playing a mental summer slide show with Diamond Rio in Concert singing "One More Day." There is Leah on my patio watering flowers in her pajamas with her little green duck sprinkling can. What a great evening when the Matthias siblings gathered in our backyard bantering as adults reminiscent of days gone by. I so loved that night when Mark and I lingered over the bonfire eating s'mores reflecting on memories and blessings. There's Leah again...we are marching, hiding, sneaking, and trying to say "Bye-Bye" to our shadows. THE END! We should have had more friends over for barbecues. We should have had more bonfires. We never got that berm planted or that storage shed built. I wish we would have taken the grandchildren to the zoo. We should have played more and worked less. I am mourning the loss of the summer season!

Today, I am reminded of the convoy of cancer feelings that emulate the change of seasons. When you first hear those words "you have cancer," you are numb and in disbelief. It is the season of shock. This season is followed by the stormy season of anger, fear, and mourning. Why me? I have never done anything to deserve this. I am so scared of what lies ahead! You mourn the loss of body parts, hair, a career, independence, intimacy; and, at times, friends. You may have regrets of unfulfilled dreams or perhaps regrets of other kinds. You mourn the lost season of normalcy. The mundane becomes devoured by testing, surgery, doctor appointments, and treatments. You long for just "one more day" of "every day life." Hopefully, all who are given a cancer diagnosis can move on to the final season–the season of acceptance. For when you enter this season, you slowly come back to life again. The once pungent air becomes filled with the sweetness of serenity and the sounds of stillness. It is a time of peace. My prayer for each and every one of you reading this is that you can keep *movin' on* with grace and with dignity to each season that God grants you. Any may you always be open to see His artistry, hear His acoustics, and smell His aromas.

Lastly, I must share that my melancholy mood has elevated to a state of elation! I received a phone call from our son Ryan this afternoon...we will have a new grandson on Friday. I can smell spring in the air, the trees are in bloom, and I see a new little bud shooting out of the ground. I'm *movin' on!*

The Pearl Moments

*I*t's Thanksgiving Day as I write this. My belly is full and my heart is satiated. As I sat in church today I couldn't help but notice a picture in our service program of an open clam shell with a pearl inside. I thought it odd at first as there were no pilgrims, turkeys, pumpkins, gourds, or corn jumping out at me. Why a clam shell and a pearl? My mind started to wonder...our hearts are much like clam shells. At times our hearts are desolately shut tight; but when a heart opens up wide, you catch a glimmer of all that is beautiful inside. Please allow me to share one of the many pearls inside of my heart today.

Several weeks ago my son Ryan and his wife Angela asked us to babysit Leah on her second birthday as they had a wedding to attend. It was a joy and a privilege to share that day with her. That morning I got her usual breakfast of toast and 'nannas ready. And then I made the best decision of my life. I decided to have coffee with a two year old! We were sitting there eating 'nannas and toast, and she was gazing out the window at the neighbor's horses. In the wonderment of a child, she asked me, "Horsies eat 'nannas and toast?" I replied, "No Leah, I think horsies eat water and hay." Then in deep conversation, she tilted her head to the side and quite seriously asked, "Cows drink milk?" And I replied, "Yes Leah, Grampa Gary's calves drink milk out of a bucket." Then she inquired what birds eat for breakfast as she saw them sitting on a bush in front of her kitchen window. I told Leah that birds eat berries, seeds, bugs, and worms. "YUCKY" was the next response! And then Leah titled her head to the side and said, "Leah happy. Oma happy too!" My response was "Yes Leah, Oma is so happy!" There was a long pause and then came the "pearl moment" from a two year old as she said, "I like Oma!" With tears streaming down my cheeks, I whispered, "I like Leah too!"

Over the past few weeks, I have opened up my heart to repeatedly pull out that gem. Why, I have asked myself? What kind of life lessons did I grasp in a one minute conversation with a two year old? That morning there was no TV, no radio, no remotes, no interruptions…it was just an innocent child and I. I looked out of a kitchen window with a two year old and have never seen the world more clearly. Leah gave me a mini refresher course in the lost art of conversation and the lost art of listening. Through the eyes of a child, I was once again reminded of all that is pure and simple.

Through the eyes of a child, I was taught how to be still to receive "pearl moments."

Thank you, Leah!

~~Oma Mary

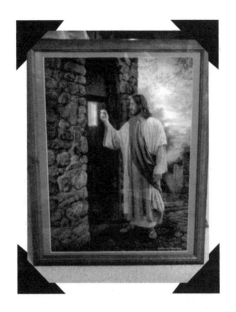

The Missing Peace

*H*ave you ever found yourself teetering on the edge of that wall; or perhaps, you have taken that great fall? Have you ever felt broken, unglued, or shattered? Has your life ever felt like a thousand pieces that could not be put together again?

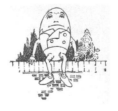

Humpty Dumpty
sat on a wall,

Humpty Dumpty
had a great fall;
All the King's horses,
and all the King's men
Could not put Humpty
together again.

All of life is full of brokenness…broken bodies, broken bank accounts, broken homes, broken family units, broken relationships, broken communication, and broken hearts. It is amidst the broken pieces that often the light shines through. It is where the missing pieces can be found. Life is a puzzle.

Please allow me to share a story of one man's brokenness and his ability to find purpose in each piece of his life. Henry is a 58 year old hardworking, witty, gentle man filled with the love of his family, his friends, and the love of Jesus. Henry is also filled with cancer. He knows that he is terminal, and yet he knows of the miracles that Jesus has performed. He knows and believes in the power of prayer. It has been a privilege for me to visit Henry and his family as he sits and shares his stories and his passion for puzzles. Henry has always had a love for puzzles, but it seems to be his sustenance these days. At times he gets very frustrated especially with "The Last Supper" puzzle. Henry would joke that it "nearly killed him." But Henry never gave up, and it is with great pride that he shares "the big picture" along with his complete puzzle repertoire. Henry explains that when he attacks a puzzle he does not look at the picture on the box–he simply takes it one piece at a time. Henry's whole family has become involved in the puzzle philosophy to the point of his daughter Shelley writing a beautiful analogy. She writes of the frustrations of that one missing piece:

"You search frantically around in hopes that the vacuum cleaner did not suck it

up, you overturn the box, chairs, tables, and rugs. There are two options 1) you find the piece and jump up and down in elation; or 2) the manufacturer screwed up and now you are left downhearted because the puzzle is incomplete. Coming from a Christian perspective and looking upon the puzzle of life…#2 can't be an option. The manufacturer is perfect. He doesn't screw up. Sometimes we feel like we are missing a piece…like life doesn't seem complete, and yet, somehow the pieces always fit together."

Henry had a farewell party a few weeks back. He wanted to say good-bye to his friends rather than have them come and bid farewell to him. Seventy-one people came to pay tribute to Henry and his family on that joyful day. Henry has all of his funeral arrangements made, his pallbearers picked out, his hymns of praise, and he has planned a parade…YES a parade. In addition to his puzzle passion, Henry has been passionate about restoring old tractors. He would like to be escorted to the cemetery by his vintage tractors. What irony that the words upon his cake on that bittersweet farewell day read, "Thank you for letting your light shine through!"

Henry achieved his goal to complete and frame a masterpiece for each of his children to hang in their homes. Yet Henry has attained a much grander goal. Shelley goes on to write,

"Not one puzzle is exactly alike…yet the goal is the same…to complete the puzzle…to see the "big picture"…to complete the task the Manufacturer has given to us. And, if we choose to display the puzzle when it is completed, we can be confident that the glue that holds us together is faith, our faith in Christ Jesus."

Are you feeling puzzled? Are you wondering how to put the pieces of your life together? What is the glue that holds it all together for you? What gives your life purpose? What makes your light shine through?

Let it shine, let it shine, let it shine!

Thank you, Henry and Shelley for giving me permission to share your story.

Addendum: *Henry has reached his goal, and the big picture is now complete. On Jan. 31, 2009, Henry was escorted to the cemetery on the back of a flat bed trailer with his best friends walking at his side and an entourage of his restored antique tractors leading the procession. It was everything he asked for and more! It was a privilege to know this man and his family.*

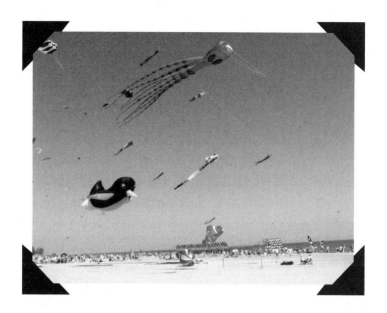

Let's Go Fly a Kite

This past week my husband and I took some vacation days. Isn't vacation time supposed to be a period of rest from work? Aren't you supposed to feel refreshed and invigorated when on vacation? At the end of the week, we were feeling accomplished about home projects that had been completed; but quite frankly, we were far from refreshed. At that point we mutually agreed to declare the next three days to be "play" days. Saturday was certainly a day to bask in the outdoors with temperatures in the 80s and a cloudless, crystal blue sky. We had heard about a community event at Neshotah Beach, Two Rivers, called "Kites Over Lake Michigan." It was free, and we didn't have to drive far; so we embarked on the first of several recreational engagements.

It turns out that this was a huge event for kite enthusiasts from all over the U.S. who share their passions of kite flying to a level of national competition! As I strolled the beach, I set my senses free not only to be refreshed but to indulge in this last summer hurrah.

My eyes were fixed to the splendor of the sky. It was a colorful image reminiscent of melted Crayola® shavings between two sheets of waxed paper. Some kites were more colorful than others, yet each one uniquely beautiful with its own shape and size. Some soared higher than others while some lifted off the ground only after the wind picked them up. Some had the gift to perform as they embellished the sky with synchronized dancing. Some hovered high above, steadfast and content to blend into the sky blue palette.

Then there were the champions of the sky's arena. Mr. Penguin sported his tux for the gala event while the gigantic blue octopus embraced the sky with his arms as though he were seven leagues under the sea. And it was no problem "finding Nemo" as this giant kite enchanted children young and old. They were truly the stars of the sky's runway and all the camera were upon them. Their faces were on the front page of the local newspapers and yet no one talked about their performance. They were the ones that soared for only a short time; and when they did, it was never too high. They had their brief moments of glory before falling flat on their backs or faces. They captured all the attention when the wind picked them up, but no one noticed them when they lay on the sandy beach.

I know you are not supposed to play favorites, but I cannot contain myself. My favorite kite was the sting-ray….he was in a league of his own. He was so colorful, so graceful, and so wise. He used the motion of his long tail to keep him from faltering. He soared higher than the penguin, the octopus, and Nemo, but not so high that he blended in with all the others. I never saw him fall…he was steadfast. He did not seem to need as much wind to make him soar. Conditions were perfect for him on that particular day, yet I wondered how he would react in less than perfect conditions.

I learned a lot about kites that day. I learned that a kite has two parts: a wing and a kite line. The kite essentially needs mooring to either a mobile or a fixed object to develop the tension in the kite line to lift it off the ground.

What kind of a kite are you? What are your mooring morals and values that keep you grounded and rooted? How do you keep your line taut? What lifts you off the ground... what makes you soar?

In Walt Disney's film "Mary Poppins," George Banks realizes that his family is more important than his job. He mends his son's kite and takes his family on a kite flying outing. Truer words were never sung!

"You can have your own set of wings
With your feet on the ground
You're a bird in a flight
With your fist holding tight
To the string of your kite."

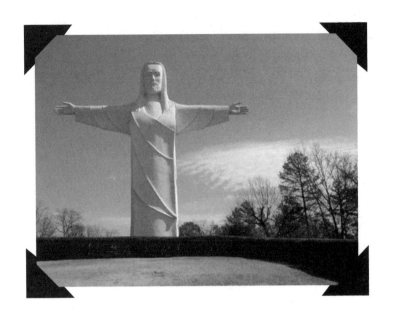

On the Wings of an Angel

Several weeks ago my twin sister and I along with our spouses spent a leisurely week in Branson, Missouri. On one of our daily excursions, we decided to explore Eureka Springs, Arkansas, home of a well-known attraction called "Christ of the Ozarks." This grandiose Jesus monument stands atop Magnetic Mountain facing west "blessing" the village of Eureka Springs. It is the third tallest Jesus sculpture in the world. Perched at an altitude of 1,500 feet, it stands 67 feet tall. Christ of the Ozarks was built by hand with more than 2 million tons of mortar and steel. Surrounding this towering image one senses a peaceful energy amidst a backdrop of serene natural beauty. As we lingered on this beautiful spring day, my sister looked through her camera's viewfinder and was awestruck. She shared what she saw…background "wings" painted by the Master artist himself. What a gift as we looked up into the sky and observed a cloud formation resembling the wings of an angel directly behind Christ's outstretched arms. It truly was an awe-huh moment. Life is full of awe-huh moments.

After our ten days of play, I once again returned to the reality show called "life." I plunged back into work, Relay meetings, and deadlines while planning Easter dinner for 20 family members. I had been procrastinating on my own ovarian cancer testing since January. As a nurse, I rationalized that with all of the recent recurrences I had seen, it was best not knowing! I woke up one Monday morning feeling physically and emotionally exhausted, not wanting to go to work. I had nothing left to give. I was feeling cancered out. I was in a funk. As I sat and had coffee with God that morning, I asked Him to help me sort my life out. If there were changes that I should make, point me in the direction. If there were commitments to relinquish, show me which ones. I went to work feeling very weary and teary knowing I had to muster up some resilience for another busy Monday. My cohorts expressed concern, and yet we had to dive in to care for all the fragile life and death situations that lie before us. As we discussed our clients, we rejoiced that one of them was turning 80 that day. Alas…someone was growing old! Florence had an ovarian cancer recurrence after 23 years and was getting chemo for her 80th birthday. I found my funk growing deeper as I calculated that this was the tenth year since my second recurrence and that maybe I would wait just a little bit longer on those tests.

I decided to wish Florence a happy birthday and offer her some "Mary hope." As I approached her, I observed a strange phenomenon. How could anyone have a smile on their face and appear happy while getting chemo on their 80th birthday? Something drew me to this beautiful soul. I pulled up a chair next to Florence as we shared our stories of cancer kinship. She proceeded to tell me about her life. In her mid 70 s, she had a wonderful job serving meals in an elderly retirement community. She loved working with the young people, could outrun them all, and even learned how to place orders on the computer. Everyone loved her...it was easy to see why. Due to health problems, she was forced to give up her job. She now spends her days as a caretaker for her two aging sisters at the Healthcare Center. She also provides rides for people needing to go to doctor's appointments. And on Friday nights, Florence and her gentleman friend can be found popping popcorn for movie night at the Healthcare Center. She talked about the importance of feeling needed and doing what we can for others. She talked about how she starts everyday with a "smile on her face" and a "song in her heart." She talked about faith and trust. She has a contagious lust for life laced with learning, laughing, and loving. Florence has a child-like spirit with wisdom that has been cultivated by 80 years of living. As I sat and listened, out of the blue I began to sob. I found myself pouring my weak and weary soul out to her. She reassured me she had times in her life where she felt the same way and put off testing in fear of the unknown. She listened, she held my hand, *she* comforted *me*...she really understood. Then she spoke, "Now, Mary, I want you to stand tall; I want you to put a smile on your face; and, I want you to put a song in your heart!"

It was more than an awe-huh moment. At that moment, I realized that God had sent a courier to deliver a powerful message. It wasn't until I looked up that I saw His outstretched arms and the wings of an angel. Florence gave me the greatest gift on her 80th birthday...she put the music back in my heart...she showed me how to soar again. I am grateful.

Addendum: *It is not smart to postpone tests. I am scheduled this week for tests with an appointment to see Dr. Matthews next week.*

God's Thumbprint

A while back I came across a research paper that my son had done many moons ago on fingerprinting. I found it interesting that no two persons have the same pattern, and the patterns remain unchanged for life. Did you know that the first recorded use of fingerprints was by the ancient Assyrians and Chinese for the signing of legal documents? I learned that the use of fingerprints for identification wasn't proposed until the late 19th century. Today, fingerprints are used to identify criminals, missing persons, and unknown deceased. Fingerprints can be found with a magic powder at crime scenes... just ask my husband, a CSI addict. They can be seen on legal documents such as birth certificates and passports and recently have played a significant role in the school systems in identifying children. And many times, fingerprints can be seen on my windows, mirrors, appliances, and coffee tables after a week-end visit from my grandchildren. Those are the ones that are hard to erase!

My son Ryan called a few days ago and asked if we could come and stay over on Saturday. Both he and Angie are in the medical field and were on call from 7:00 p.m. until 7:00 a.m. They needed someone to be there with the children in the event that they both got called in to work. They decided to take advantage of our visit and headed out with their pagers to attend a Christmas gathering that evening. What a gift…time alone with the "grands," as I call them.

Before I can move ahead, I must go back. Ben was born with a large red raised birthmark on his belly. They were told it would fade and diminish in time. Leah, their first child, found Ben's birthmark quite disturbing; and so her mom simply explained, "It is God's thumbprint on Ben." Leah came to look upon this as a special insignia. That night as I changed Ben's diaper, we discussed his birthmark. She quizzically asked, "Why do boys have thumbprints and not girls?" It was purely by the grace of God that I had an answer, "You have one too Leah, only yours can't be seen. Your thumbprint is on your heart. When Ben's goes away, it will be on his heart too." WHEW… got through that one with an image and a thought that seemed to satisfy her three year old wise soul. That is until it came to bedtime when after prayers, hugs, and numerous attempts of delay she looked at me and queried, "Why is Ben's thumbprint on the outside and why is mine on the inside?" And then I prayed, "God give me an answer quickly!" In my ineptness, I sighed, "Sometimes Dads and Moms and Pappas and Omas don't have the answers. Sometimes you just have to wait and ask Jesus! Leah was satisfied at that point or perhaps just too sleepy to want to know more. She drifted off to sleep.

I sat in awe that night as I reflected on our discussion. Because of a mother's beautiful and simple explanation of something rather unsightly, a child looked at a birthmark as a special gift from God. I think Leah was actually feeling somewhat slighted that no one could see her thumbprint.

Haven't all of our lives been marked with something unsightly? What is the birthmark that afflicts your life? Is yours on the outside? Perhaps it's your bald head...the crown of cancer. Maybe your physical scars are the wrath of disease or the result of an injury. Or were you marked from birth with a disability or a cognitive deficit? Perhaps your unsightly birthmark is on the inside where no one can see your affliction. Why are some people challenged with mental illness, chemical dependency, phobias, eating disorders, depression, and anxiety?

All of life is full of questions that have no answers. I don't know why some sufferings are on the outside and why some are on the inside, but I am certain of one thing. I was given an epiphany by a three year old child. We all have the ability to transform life's birthmarks into God's thumbprints. What comfort in knowing that His pattern is one of a kind and remains unchanged for all of eternity. The next time you find yourself questioning a happening in your life, pull out your magnifying glass. Learn to recognize His fingerprints.

"Now faith is being sure of what we hope for
and certain of what we do not see."
~~Hebrews 11:1

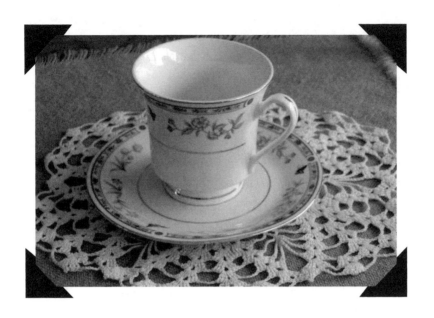

Hazie & Albert

by Jayne Purchatzke

*O*ne Monday in early spring, one of my dear cohorts presented me with a
Shopko bag and simply said, "I have something for you." Inside the bag was
something gingerly wrapped in layers of paper and bubble wrap. I peeled back the
layers to unfold a delicate teacup and saucer with butterflies and flowers encircling
the edges. As I proceeded to express my sentiments of gratitude, Jayne presented
me with the real gift...the story of two people's lives that I never even knew. Here
is how the story unfolded as told by my friend Jayne.

I'm afraid I don't know much about these two except to say
that they were colorfully intriguing and wonderful people. Albert was
originally from England but came to the United States to attend school

out East. I believe his parents were well off and could afford to send him to the U.S. Albert had a strong interest and love of nature. What he loved most were butterflies. Albert knew all there was to know about them. Hazel, who was known to most as "Hazie," was from out East. Hazie went to a local college to become a teacher. It was there that she met her beloved Albert.

Albert and Hazie dated during their college years and married shortly after graduation. Albert taught at several different colleges throughout his career while Hazie taught grade school. They had no children. During their summers, Albert taught Hazie all he knew about butterflies. She came to love them as much as he did. They traveled extensively during time off to study different species of butterflies and to enjoy the many different cultures they encountered.

When Albert and Hazie retired, they moved to a very rural area of Iola, Wisconsin. The house was old and small, and they had a barn on their property. They loved the area because it was natural and full of milkweed. Albert found pleasure in building mesh boxes. He and Hazie would then set out to pick bunches of milkweed loaded with caterpillars and place them in vases inside the mesh boxes. They would sit back and "watch the magic happen." After eating the milkweed, the caterpillars would crawl up the side of the mesh boxes, hang upside down, and turn into chrysalis. I remember as a child being in Albert and Hazie's house once. Mesh boxes were everywhere! I thought they were crazy but was too young at the time to appreciate the magic in their madness. They loved releasing their butterflies. It was a sight they never tired of. Albert and Hazie also had an extensive garden. A weed wouldn't dare grow in it. Every afternoon at 4:00 p.m., the two would sit in their garden, admire their flowers, watch their butterflies, and sip tea. One afternoon, Albert surprised Hazie with a pretty wrapped package. He gave her a cup and saucer with butterflies dancing on it. She used it everyday thereafter.

Albert died a few years back and was buried in England.

Hazie kept on raising butterflies at the young age of 92 plus years. She refused to go into a nursing home. After Albert's death, whenever she would speak of him, she'd begin with "my dear beloved Albert, God rest his soul." Hazie endearingly loved her Albert. Hazie died sometime in early 2006 and was buried in England next to her "dear beloved Albert."

My sister and I vaguely knew Hazie and Albert from our childhood and into our teen years. They were friends of our grandparents. One day in August of 2005, I visited my sister at work in the veterinarian's office. I took my pictures of Relay for Life along to show my sister the photos of the live butterfly release. She said she had to stop at Hazie's home to pick up her dog, bring it into the vet to take a look at, and then take it back. Hazie was unable to drive any longer. My sister and I went to Hazie's house...she remembered us as Marion's granddaughters. We sat with her as she was having afternoon tea with her butterfly cup. We had a hard time leaving. I admired her cup and saucer. She said, "My dear beloved Albert, God rest his soul, surprised me with it years ago. He gave me a pretty wrapped gift for no reason. I've used it everyday since." She inquired what my sister and I were doing with ourselves. I said that I was very active with the American Cancer Society's Relay for Life. She said she heard of it but didn't know what it was all about. I ran to my sister's car to get photos of the Relay event. I especially explained to her about the awesome butterfly release and the significance of it at the closing ceremony. I knew if anyone would appreciate it, she would! She loved it. I also spoke of my friend Mary Matthias who orchestrated the idea. I mentioned to her that Mary had dealt with ovarian cancer twice and showed her a picture of Mary and of the butterflies being released. She was amazed that anyone could survive cancer twice in a lifetime. Hazie never knew Mary at all but was impressed at how hard Mary must have fought to live. She said, "Mary is a very strong young lady."

Last week a young lawyer, who drove quite a distance, showed up at the veterinary clinic in Iola with a package. It was given to my sister with instructions that it was to be delivered to Mary Matthias. My friend Mary had made an impression on someone she didn't even know. Hazie willed Mary her butterfly cup and saucer. My sister brought it home so that one day Mary can pass it on.

A sincere and heartfelt thank you to my friend Jayne for so eloquently piecing this story together for me to share.

It humbles me to tears when I hold that teacup and saucer in my hand for I am holding such a personal and delicate piece of two lives that I never knew. My treasured gift safely hangs above my living room shelf as a constant reminder of the intricate matter in which all of our lives are woven together. One day I will pass it on, along with my own butterfly story, and the story of Hazie and Albert...God rest their beloved souls.

Note from Tim in TLC newsletter: A wonderful story indeed! The lesson I take from this beautiful story is that we must do what we must do. We must fight the good fight ,and live the good life not for our own benefit, but to be an example and positive influence for others! All of us, with or without cancer, have the opportunity to make this world a better place and enhance the lives of those around us...family members, friends, neighbors and strangers. Thank you Mary, Jayne, Hazie, and Albert!

Saved by the Bell

*J*ust last week I heard an old, yet familiar saying chanted by one of our Cancer Care Center patients, "Saved by the bell." The origin of that quote was certainly reminiscent of school days when the recess bell or the end of class bell resounded saving me from a boring lecture, an additional assignment, a question that had me squirming, or perhaps it saved me from a geometry or chemistry quandary. Back then, "saved by the bell" meant I was on my way...on my way to the playground, on my way to another class, or perhaps on my way to meet my boyfriend at his locker.

At the Holy Family Memorial Cancer Care Center, bells can be heard ringing throughout the halls on any given day. Not only can you hear bells and acclamations of applause; but if you listen closely, you will hear teardrops falling. In recent months, staff members of the radiation and medical oncology units at the Cancer Care Center pondered on a way to celebrate our patients completing their arduous course of chemotherapy or extensive radiation treatments. We wanted to find a profound way to recognize and validate the significance of that day with our patients and their caregivers. During this time of brainstorming, I was approached by Dr. Shariff regarding a show he had seen on TV called "Houston Medical." He went on to explain that there was a woman named Marnie who upon completion of her treatment for pancreatic cancer had tolled a bell while reading a poem of victory. He added, "It was really neat, Mary...you should implement that into the Cancer Care Center."

Upon completion of treatment, each survivor is now invited to gather around the bell with their team of caregivers for a brief but bittersweet ceremony. With heads held high and tears filled with emotion, they ring the bell. For those sitting in the chemo bay, this observation has turned into a tangible goal. I have heard many patients declare, "I am going to ring the bell!" Unfortunately not everyone gets to ring the bell, but recently one of our patients shed a whole new light on the bell. Her cancer was not responding to treatment so she prayerfully and peacefully decided to end treatment. Her request that day was to ring the bell. That truly marked a day of celebration...she had at last found peace.

My most cherished bell-ringing story is about Fran. Upon discharge from the hospital, Fran requested to come through the CCC and ring the bell. She was entering the hospice program and going home to die. Fran entered the chemo bay being pushed in her wheelchair by her husband who is also a cancer survivor. She was surrounded by her usual entourage of family and friends. As she rang the bell, a DNR (do not resuscitate) bracelet was placed on her wrist; and she proclaimed, "There! I am now on my way!" She said she was going home to lie in her hospital bed by the window, watch her birds, and surround herself with family and friends. Never did the bell toll so well for these are the words proudly proclaimed:

Ringing Out

(As seen on "Houston Public" television show)

Ring this bell
Three times well
A toll to clearly say
This treatment's done
My course is run
And I am on my way

*I*n memory of their special moment, each patient is given a laminated card with an angel pin attached that echoes the words above. After emotional farewells, hugs, and tears, they are sent "on their way." Indeed it is the prayer of our entire Cancer Care Center team that many will be *"saved by the bell."*

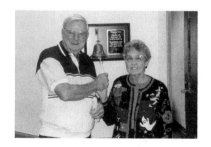

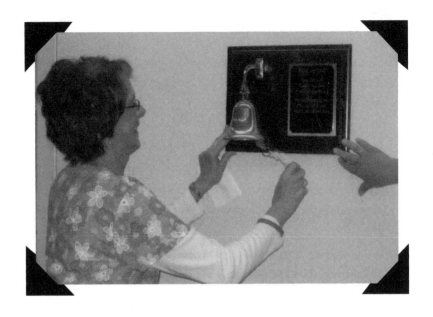

My 10 Year Cancerversary

*M*ay 29, 2006, marked my 10 year cancerversary from the time I was first diagnosed. I pondered on how I could carry this celebration into my work day. It was important for me to share this day with my co-workers as well as with our patients. I decided to ring the bell.

These are the words I humbly proclaimed:

> Ring this bell
> Ten times well
> Ten tolls to clearly say
> All praise and glory be
> for what He has done for me
> I'm alive, I'm alive
> What a wonderful day.

On that special day, my sister Carol surprised me and my friends with a catered in meal for lunch and a beautiful spring bouquet of flowers. It truly was a memorable and wonderful day.

My Ovarian Idol

I am not a poet by any means, but I have taken a few writing classes. During one of my classes I wrote this poem about Fran. She had ovarian cancer. Fran always created hoopla and brought jocularity into the Chemo Bay. She left fingerprints on our souls in the way that she lived and in the way that she died. She endured a lot; she was endeared by many.

Frances

There was something exceptional about her
from the moment she first sauntered through the doors.

A place of suffering, where lives are mutated by mutated cells converted into a sanctuary of joy and jocularity by her mere presence.

Images of her linger like an exotic fragrance.

Conversations begin and end with her name.

Like confetti sprinkles on a cake, she was an array of color.

With her red crass curls, she mirthfully ministered to the soul pain of her spectators.

"Billy" was her knight and her rock, yet she chided, "He is still a work in progress."

She filled the room with many hues but rarely did you see her wear the color blue.

Nothing moved except her foot steps as she won the attention of breathless crowds

In her youth, she was a tightrope walker.

Perhaps that is how she learned to master the fine line between hope and despair.

I have combed the crevices of my mind to find a place where I can see her again.

In my apocalypse I have found her.

It is a place filled with rides that take you up and down and around and around.

On roller coasters, she rides with me, my faithful phantom companion.

The sound of her voice articulates in the music of her memories.

Like lemonade and cotton candy...

She captivates the bittersweet palate of my life.

She was a one woman act...a legacy without replacement.

"I am on my way," she whispered as silently as her disease.

Fran was the diva of a malady that destroyed her life.

Cancer transcended her soul.

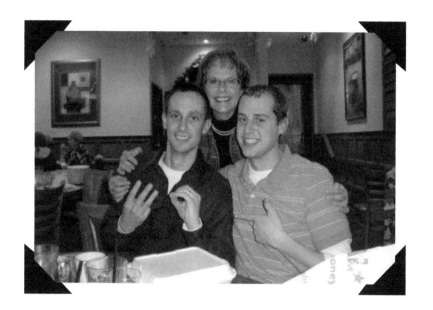

Luke's Story

As I begin to put closure to my book, I find that there is within me a compelling call to share one final story. I have been asking myself why? After 11 years, why am I feeling the need to tell this particular story? It is a story of profound pain manifested into an amazing revelation. It is a story that has taken me 11 years to process. It is my son's story.

Before I sat down to tell this story today, I called Luke up to ask his permission to share it. In his wisdom he said, "I think the story needs to be told because it has now gone full circle." He went on to explain that his experience was similar to mine in that he too needed to feel the pain before he could feel the joy. He confessed that it had taken him many years to process his life-altering event. Luke's story changed his entire life. What started out as a beautiful, fun, summer evening nearly ended in a double tragedy? We almost lost both of our sons. Here is how the story vividly unfolds.

August 28, 1999

It was a beautiful summer evening. I donned my wig, my new dress, and some dancing shoes. I remember feeling pretty attractive that night (something I had not felt for a while). We were headed out for an evening away from cancer. We had been invited to my cousin's daughter's wedding. I was anticipating a fun evening of catch up conversation with my cousins, good food, and some dancing with my husband. I was feeling very lighthearted as I said goodbye to Ryan and Luke. Ryan was home from college, and it filled my heart with such joy to see them throwing the football around in the back yard and grilling out together. I remember thinking what a gift it was to have two sons who got along so well.

As we arrived at the reception, we were warmly greeted by genuinely caring family members and friends inquiring on my current state of health. I was out of my two year remission and undergoing chemotherapy once again. I was grateful for everyone's love and concern, but I was silently wishing for a cancer free night. I remember being so happy that my taste buds were back to normal as I savored the food. I was about to dive into a delectable dessert when I was paged to come to the front desk of the hotel for a phone call. I found that a little odd as I did not leave my sons with a phone number. It was Dr. Shariff on the phone and these were his words, "Mary, you need to get home immediately. Your son was electrocuted tonight and your other son relentlessly risked his own life to save his brother." We raced home not knowing what led up to this near fatal event. I pleaded with God all the way to the hospital to spare my sons' lives.

As we arrived in the Emergency Room, we were met by a nurse who profoundly affirmed, "We witnessed a miracle tonight. People don't usually live through this kind of a thing." As she guided us to the intensive care unit, we began to piece together what had occurred. Luke had gone into the garage to plug in the boom box, and he did not come back out. Ryan heard him yell out but thought he was "dorking around." After a short time, Ryan went in to check up on him and found him down on the ground totally contracted, blue, and not breathing. There was something faulty with the metal power box that he plugged the boom box into. It is the kind of voltage that attaches itself to you and does not throw you away from it. The box landed on his right chest. Ryan had the wits about him to know he had to get it off of him. He grabbed the cord and pulled the box off of Luke knowing that he was exposing himself to the same current that was shocking his brother. He then ran into the house to call 911. As he returned and was ready to start CPR, Luke gasped and started to breathe again.

That night as we entered the Intensive Care Unit, I did not know who to console first—my wise and courageous son Ryan who, by the grace of God, was unharmed yet emotionally traumatized or my son Luke whose body had been physically traumatized. I remember going into the bathroom that night, taking my wig off, and splashing cold water on my face. I looked in the mirror and started to scream at God, *"I don't care what you do to me, but leave my sons alone."* I was so angry at God. I almost lost both of my sons! I remember people telling me to be grateful because it *didn't* happen. How could I possibly be grateful? Ryan was psychologically scarred. Luke was angry, not eating, and severely depressed because he could not play football. We were concerned about the long term ramifications of this kind of voltage on Luke's body. Mark was beating himself up about the wiring in the garage, and I was in the middle of the wraths of chemotherapy. How dare anyone tell me to be grateful? It wasn't until Luke shared with us his "near death experience" that the healing began and the anger began to dissipate.

The following is Luke's soulful recapture of his experience:

"I remember all I could see was white. I had the sensation of flying, flying really fast. It was a very comforting and warm feeling. It was not scary at all. While I had the flying sensation and could only see white, I remember hearing voices that sounded like when you walk into a crowded auditorium. There were all kinds of voices, but I couldn't hear one voice above the others. I felt like I was flying above a football field. I remember all of a sudden I could faintly make out one voice above the rest. I couldn't make anything out of it at first, but it slowly got louder and louder. I felt as if I was flying toward the voice. As I got closer and closer to the voice, it kept escalating until all the other voices were drowned out. Someone was yelling my name. That is when I remember opening my eyes for a brief second and seeing Ryan above me. I closed my eyes again and reopened them. Every blink I took got shorter and shorter; and as I came to, I saw Ryan above me yelling my name. I remember looking at Ryan thinking he looked worse than I felt. As I was getting loaded onto a stretcher and into the ambulance, I turned and asked Ryan if this meant we couldn't play catch anymore. I saw a bit of relief in his eyes, probably thinking I was going to be all right. Overall, that whole time when I was out was one of the most peaceful and wonderful feelings I can remember—complete serenity. It is a thought that I often come back to and try to recapture whenever I am stressed out or having a bad day. While I cannot relive the serenity of that brief moment in time, I am comforted by and confident in knowing that death is not an end but just a new beginning."

Why do I share this with you after 11 years? It's because I think too often we can't move beyond the anger of chance events to see God's plan unfold. Three years after this event, I came home from work one day and Luke was sitting at the counter looking like the cat that had swallowed the canary. I asked him, "What's up with you?" He shared that when he was cutting lawn that day he had a light bulb moment. He said that he went to his college and changed all of his classes around. He went on to say, "I figure God didn't keep me alive to sit behind a desk and move papers around all day. I am going to be a teacher."

Luke is now the most caring, loving 7th grade Social Studies teacher. Ryan is in the medical field working in the cardiac cath lab where he continues to help save lives. They have a special brotherly bond that is far deeper than blood. Today, I asked Luke what he had learned from processing this life changing event. He responded, "What happened to me made me the person that I am today. I am much more appreciative, and I like to think I have my priorities straight. My near death experience was much like yours Mom."

Carpe Diem ✝ Seize the Day

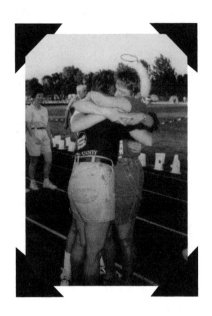

My Living Legacy
How to Embrace Life

1) *A*lways be patient and gentle. Set realistic goals so that you have something to work for and look forward to. Celebrate reaching those goals.

2) Get passionate about something. It will keep your heart happy and hope filled.

3) Learn to recognize when fear, worry, and stress are destroying your hope. Regroup and gather back that which saves you. And then quiet your soul to listen to the whisperings of the Holy Spirit.

4) Remember that often it's our limitations that send our imaginations and creativity soaring. When the body is not working up to its potential, let your mind and spirit take over.

5) Trust that hope will always keep you afloat. Breath it, pray it, and embrace it.

6) Be at peace with yourself, with others, and with your God. Only then can you live a life of harmony.

7) Live all your life preparing to leave behind a generous donation of love. What greater contribution can you make to society?

8) Be open to life around you. Pay attention to people and circumstances. Learn to identify God's fingerprints on your life.

9) Listen to the gentle raindrops as well as the rolling thunder. Hope can be subtle and not always dramatic.

10) Honor your tears. They are the holy water of hope and healing. Golda Meir once said, "Those who don't know how to weep with their whole heart don't know how to laugh either."

Finding the "ancer" in cancer

Charlie, it would not be fair to end *my* story without bringing it back to *your* story. YES, I do believe there will be cows in Heaven…in fact, I think there may be a herd waiting for you when you arrive.

Charlie's simple query is characteristic of the countless daunting questions that evolve when given a life-altering diagnosis. It has been through the guidance of a team of health care professionals, my family, my friends, and my loving God that I have come to find the "ancer" in cancer.

In one of my early journal entries I wrote…

January 22, 2001

"Cancer has been my daily companion for four years and eight months now. Sometimes it is my friend because it has led me to people and places beyond my dreams. It has made me see, touch, taste, smell, and feel a crispness and a depth that I never knew existed in life. It has made me dream, believe, and reach! It has taught me how to savor each sweet bite of today. Cancer has re-defined faith, love, trust, and HOPE again and again! It has bestowed bountiful blessings in my life and those who rally around me as cheerleaders in a pep band. Cancer will be my companion until the end–I just have to learn to befriend it."

In all of life, God gives us journeys and wisdom to be found.
Remember to return Home, for that is where stories abound!

♥

Live to Learn
Learn to Love
Love to Live

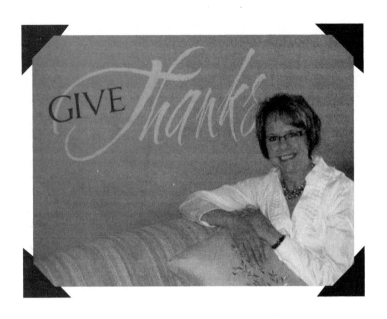

About the Author...

...*I*'s Not About Me!

Self-publishing this book has been an incredible learning experience. Throughout it all, my husband of almost 35 years has been such a wise and supportive soul; to him I *give thanks!*

I guess this is the page where I'm supposed to share my credentials and proclaim any fame that I may have. Well this page is not about *me*; it's about *my God!* He is my eminence! Because of Him, I know that I will spend an eternity in heaven. Indeed I do give thanks—for every day—for every grace-filled moment—for the truth that sets me free!

"Surely it is God who saves me...I will trust in him and not be afraid..."
First Song of Isaiah